HOW TO
BATTLE
SEASICKNESS

100 TIPS
TO HELP YOU GET
YOUR SEA LEGS

MICHELLE SEGREST

HOW TO BATTLE SEASICKNESS

100 TIPS TO HELP YOU GET YOUR SEA LEGS

BY MICHELLE SEGREST

eBook (ISBN 978-1-7346757-3-3)
Paperback (ISBN 978-1-0880-6215-9)
Hardcover (ISBN 978-8-440850-4-2)

www.navigatecontent.com/sailing-adventure-blog

Disclaimer

HOW TO BATTLE SEASICKNESS
100 Tips to Help You Get Your Sea Legs

Michelle Segrest has experienced epic battles with seasickness while sailing the world on a 43-foot steel ketch with only a two-person crew. She has learned that beginners are not the only ones who suffer from the phenomenon. Since the beginning of time, humans have battled their way through seasickness—even experienced captains and seasoned sailors. With a small crew and passages that often extend for weeks, it is important to learn how to function and fight your way through the incredibly uncomfortable symptoms and effects of seasickness.

In this book, Michelle combines exhaustive research with a few of her own grueling experiences. Most important, she offers 100 proven tips to help you understand the phenomenon, prevent it, and battle your way through it. Some of these methods are pharmaceutical, some are natural, some are psychological. She includes advice from doctors, sailors, mariners, fishermen, and seasoned boat captains in addition to her advice after trying possibly every so-called remedy herself.

You don't have to be sailing offshore blue waters in a small sailboat to benefit from the knowledge shared in this book. These tips will help you whether you are in a sailboat, motorboat, fishing boat, kayak, canoe, car, airplane, or cruise ship.

There is no cure for seasickness. However, this book will help you find your sea legs and battle your way through it.

Table of Contents

INTRODUCTION

In my experience, there are two kinds of sailors. Those who get seasick, and those who lie about it.

There is no cure for seasickness. However, it can be helpful to learn ways to prevent it and how to cope with it.

For some of us, the wretched phenomenon is a given every time we go to sea. At some point you just accept that it's going to happen. It can be minor, or it can be severe. But it will affect some of us to some degree on every passage. Even sitting at anchorage or in a marina, some of us tend to get queasy at times from the motion. I have personally suffered from it so severely that even the activity of researching and writing this book has made me a little queasy at times. I don't just remember what it's like to be seasick—at times, I can still feel it!

For others, the seasickness strikes less frequently. The bouts can be shorter and manageable, and perhaps they only show up in heavy offshore conditions or for other specific reasons.

An experienced sailor once told me that it's all about tolerances. For him, he was fine until the waves reached three meters, then he generally became seasick. But in sailing conditions with less than three-meter waves, he was fine. We will spend more than a few pages diving deeply into the fascinating psychology of seasickness.

While some sailors only suffer mild seasickness and infrequently, for some, the debilitating effects can last nonstop for several straight days, as it did for me in September 2018 while crossing the Bay of Biscay in a 43-foot steel ketch.

At some point in time, I believe that every sailor experiences some level of seasickness—even if they don't suffer as severely as I do. Experience can help. Preventive measures can help. And one thing is certain—nothing is as awful and debilitating as the first time. There are ways to manage the uneasiness and to quell its effects. But let's be clear—there is no sure-fire cure.

Seasickness is a fascinating phenomenon. I am ultimately intrigued by it when I am not experiencing it. Therefore, I have studied it deeply and intently. I have researched and tried almost all the so-called cures—chemical, physical, natural, and psychological.

I decided to write this book to share with you my exhaustive research as well as some of my experiences and the experiences of fellow sailors around the globe. It's a common topic among sailors, and every experience with seasickness is different.

I've been sailing since 2013. For a year (August 2018 to August 2019) I sailed some of the world's most challenging passages on a 43-foot, steel ketch, *Seefalke*, with only a two-person crew (and a couple of beagles, who also experienced motion sickness at times). Even with different levels of sailing experience, both the seasoned skipper and I battled our way through seasickness many times during the voyage. It's a necessity. With only a two-person crew and passages that often extend for weeks at a time, it is important to learn how to function and fight your way through the incredibly uncomfortable symptoms and effects of seasickness.

While fighting my own battles, I was desperate to find something—*anything*—that would help me. This is another reason I wanted to write this book. Hopefully it will help you if you are a victim of this horrible phenomenon.

In this book, I combine all of my exhaustive research on the topic and share some grueling first-hand experiences with explicit detail. After reading some of my stories, you will know what it feels like to be seasick. Most important, I offer **100 Tips to Help You Get Your Sea Legs**—to help you understand the phenomenon, to help you prevent it, and to help you battle it.

Some of my methods are pharmaceutical, some are natural, some are psychological. Some of them are proven tips and tricks from my own experience and some are from the experiences of fellow sailors and boating enthusiasts from around the globe.

I also share a few tips that helped our four-legged crew members—beagles Cap'n Jack and Scout. And yes, dogs and other animals also can experience seasickness.

I was inspired to write this book based on all the comments and responses I frequently receive on my online blog, **"How to Get Your Sea Legs"** (Segrest, 2018, 2019, 2020, 2021). It's an award-winning blog that chronicles my sailing adventures that include graphic and detailed battles with seasickness. Revised versions of some of my blogs are included in this book.

I want to stress that I am a sailor, and I am a journalist. But I am NOT a doctor. I am not a health care professional of any kind, and I don't claim to be one or pretend to be one. In this book, I share some information about pharmaceuticals that I have tried (even though they all failed for me, they may help you). I encourage you to consult a doctor before trying any medication to battle seasickness or motion sickness. I do not recommend ANY of the pharmaceutical remedies for seasickness. I can only tell you that they exist so that you can consult your doctor to discuss whether they may be an option for you.

The methods that have helped me the most are natural and psychological. By sharing my specific experiences and my extensive research, I hope that you will understand that you are not alone, and that there are some great tips and techniques that will help you!

You don't have to be sailing in blue waters hundreds of miles offshore in a small sailboat to benefit from the knowledge shared in this book. I use the terms "seasickness" and "motion sickness" interchangeably, and these tips will help you whether you are in a sailboat, motorboat, fishing boat, battleship, rowboat, canoe, kayak, cruise ship, airplane, spaceship, or automobile.

There is no cure for seasickness.

However, this book will help you find your sea legs so you can battle your way through it.

CHAPTER 1

You Never Forget Your First Time

As we left the wind shadow of the island of Rønne, Denmark, in May 2016, the contents of my belly began to boil as the 30-knot gusts and 3-meter waves rocked our 24-foot sailboat, *Toja*, from side to side, up and down, back and forth. The queasiness was overwhelming—much worse than the flu, or food poisoning, or even a harsh hangover.

My head felt like it would split in two while the sweat poured down my face, even though the air was chilled at about 28-degrees Fahrenheit.

I could feel my color turn a pall green, as my eyesight began to blur.

I was sitting on the high side of the cockpit as *Toja* was heeling at about 25 degrees. I had just put on my life vest over my heavy winter coat. I looked at the captain and began to quiver. I could feel the contents of my belly rising to my throat.

"I'm about to lose it," I heard myself say in a surprisingly calm monotone.

Then I quickly moved to the low side and emptied my insides with brutal force. I heard the D-ring clamp into place as the captain strapped me into the cockpit with a safety harness to keep me from falling into the cold waters of the Baltic Sea.

Or, perhaps, it was to keep me from throwing myself overboard, which is exactly what I wanted to do.

I stayed in that position for the next 10 hours until there was nothing left to exit my body but foul-tasting, burning, boiling acid, and blood sprinkled with bits and pieces of my stomach lining.

I finally found the strength to let go of the rail and lie flat on my back on the cockpit floor. My head was right next to the locker that contained the diesel tanks, and even though the engine was not running, I could smell the fumes. This didn't help my situation, but I couldn't move. I was paralyzed.

The captain wasn't feeling well either, but he had to push through. He had no choice. There was nothing I could do to help him, and frankly I didn't care whether we made it to our destination or sank. At least one of us needed to sail the ship.

I stayed in this position for 10 straight hours.

I could feel the dehydration set in as my calves and back began to spasm with knotty muscle cramps. I asked the captain when the nightmare would end.

"When the boat stops," he said in his usual stoic, matter-of-fact way.

"How long until that happens?" I asked with sincere and desperate anticipation.

"Oh, not much longer," he said calmly. "We are almost there. Only another four hours to go."

"FOUR MORE HOURS!" *There was no way I could continue to feel like this for FOUR MORE HOURS!*

I decided to try and work my way down the three steps into the cabin. I slithered like a snake, backward, head first, very slowly down the steps, trying to hold back the impending retching.

With hardly any hydration, I couldn't believe I needed to pee. But after sailing for four hours, then hanging over the side of the rail for another 2 hours, then lying on the cockpit floor for 10 hours, I definitely needed to pee. I managed to get my pants down and slowly made my way to the head. I released the last few drops of fluid in my body but didn't have the energy to pull up my pants.

I collapsed flat on my back on the bunk, pants still down around my ankles. Then I passed out, completely surrendering to my first-ever bout with seasickness.

Four hours later, we entered the channel to Karliskrona, Sweden. The rocking boat and my dilapidated body had calmed as we entered the marina.

All of a sudden, I felt fine. Seriously. I felt just fine. Just like that.

I jumped up from the bunk as if I had somewhere exciting to go. I pulled up my pants and made my way to the deck. I prepared the mooring lines, secured all the fenders, grabbed the boat hook, and helped the captain safely moor *Toja*.

I ate a few nibbles of bread and drank an entire 1.5-liter bottle of water in what seemed like one gulp. I looked up at the captain and confidently stated, "I still want to sail. I'll find a way to beat this." Then I crashed.

The next morning, I asked the captain if we could cruise around Karliskrona a bit. I wanted to immediately get back my sea legs. I wanted to be sure that the 20-hour passage filled with vile, retching misery would not be the last memory I ever had of sailing.

At the time, I had been sailing for four years, but this was my first experience with seasickness.

It wouldn't be the last.

TIPS FROM CHAPTER 1

- Strap yourself securely in the cockpit to prevent falling out of the boat. (Or to prevent throwing yourself overboard, which may be what you feel like doing.)
- Stay away from areas with strong smells, like the locker containing the diesel tanks.
- Try to stay hydrated to prevent dehydration and muscle cramps.
- Try to eat something, even if you throw it back up. Try to digest some calories.
- Remember that the effects of seasickness most likely will not stop until the motion stops, so accept this and try not to panic.
- Don't watch the clock. Try to focus on something else, if at all possible, so you don't focus on how much time is still to go on the passage.
- If possible, lie flat on your back in the cabin and try to sleep (sometimes this is not possible if you are sailing with a small crew).
- Get back out there as soon as possible so you don't lose your nerve later. You don't want this to be your last-ever memory of sailing.

CHAPTER 2

What is Seasickness and Motion Sickness?

I think it's possible that until you truly experience seasickness, you can't really say that you know what it is. Not really. You can say you've been queasy, or that you felt a bit dizzy. But let me assure you that when you truly experience seasickness, you'll know it!

According to experts, seasickness (also called *mal de mer*) is the reaction of your body's inner ear balance system to the unfamiliar motion of the ship. The movement of the ship causes stress on the balancing portion of the brain. Your brain sees things on the ship such as walls and furniture and instinctively knows from past experience that they are supposed to be still.

But when you are on a boat, everything is in motion. The air is moving. The sea beneath you is moving. And yes, everything on the ship is moving at least a little bit—even when you think everything is safely secured.

Since all these items that are supposed to be still are actually moving with the sea and the ship, the inner ear gets stressed and confused and nausea sets in.

Seasickness often disappears within a few days, even without treatment. The brain eventually adjusts to this new environment, and the sufferer gets his or her "sea legs." For me, it's usually about three days of seasickness, then I begin to feel fine for the rest of the passage. One unfortunate aspect of long trans-ocean voyages is that once you reach your destination, it may take a while for you to adjust to being on land again. (Garrison, 2019)

When John Konrad was asked the question, "What is the definition of misery?" his answer was simple—Seasickness. He says he only experienced it once, and describes it this way:

"I was cooking lasagna in the galley of a 37-foot sailboat racing upwind in 20-foot swells when the kerosene lamp broke. Taken separately, the confined space, heavy rolls, the smell of lasagna, and kerosene never bothered me much, but the combination of all four proved insurmountable. Luckily, I just went topside and waited for the cabin to air out, but the 60 seconds it took me to escape were pure misery. The single worst aspect of seasickness is not being able to stop it. Seasickness on a boat is never a major problem as it's usually only a short trip to the nearest harbor but, in the middle of the ocean, your only option is to wait until the seas calm down. This can take days." (Konrad, 2016)

Is Motion Sickness Different from Seasickness?

Sometimes the best prevention is knowledge so, to answer the question, motion sickness is a generic term for the discomfort and associated vomiting induced by a variety of motion conditions aboard ships, aircraft, vehicles, on swings or amusement park rides, in zero gravity environments (e.g. space), and elevators.

Actually, the term "motion sickness" is somewhat of a misnomer from two perspectives. First, it can be induced in the absence of motion, for example during a virtual reality simulation, and secondly, sickness implies that it is a type of disease, when in fact it is a perfectly normal response of a healthy individual without any functional disorders (Benson, 1999). Although the symptoms and physiological responses are consistent for all motions, seasickness varies with the individual. (Konrad, 2016)

Signs of Seasickness

According to the website Dizziness and Balance, motion sickness (also called seasickness) is the nausea, disorientation and fatigue that can be induced by head motion. The first sign is usually pallor (a pale appearance). Yawning, restlessness, and a cold sweat forming on the upper lip or forehead often follow. As symptoms build, an upset stomach, fatigue or drowsiness may occur. The final stages are characterized by nausea and vomiting.

Motion sickness is a general term. It can be subdivided into sickness due to visual stimulation, due to vestibular stimulation, and occasionally, forms occur associated with somatosensory stimulation (e.g. treadmill sickness), or head-on-neck motion (e.g. cervical vertigo). By far the most common subgroup are pure visual sensitivity—usually called "visual dependence." In visual dependence, people become sick due to visual motion (such as going to a movie). (Hain, 2020)

According to the Centers for Disease Control, nearly 100% of us have—or will—succumb to seasickness on rough waters. Scientists have a fancy name for this malady—kinetosis—and it's an age-old problem. (Erskine, 2019)

Think of it as a battle of the senses. Seasickness occurs when one part of your balance-sensing system (your inner ear, eyes, and sensory nerves) senses that your body is moving, but the other parts do not. For example, if you're in the cabin of a moving vessel, your inner ear may sense the motion of waves, but your eyes don't detect any movement. This sensory mismatch confuses your brain, and in turn, you feel sick.

Symptoms of seasickness run the gamut from dry mouth, cold sweats, dizziness and drowsiness to mild headaches, nausea and vomiting. In other words, pure misery. (Boater, 2018)

History of Motion Sickness

Motion sickness has been around as long as there has been people and motion. It was well known to the Greeks and Romans. Around 300 AD the Chinese described "Cart-influence" and "Ship-influence." Admiral Nelson, the British naval hero who first went to sea at the age of 12, was a chronic sufferer. (Timothy C. Hain, 2019)

Ancient Greeks referred to seasickness as the "plague of the sea," and famous sufferers through the ages include Christopher Columbus, Admiral Horatio Lord Nelson and Charles Darwin. (Guru, 2021)

Even the most seasoned mariners can fall prey to seasickness. Medical reports submitted by crews after the 2012 Newport to Bermuda race included 54 cases of seasickness. (Jeffrey Wisch, 2021) And according to a *Yachting World* survey of 450 sailors taking part in a 2015 ARC transatlantic rally, 26% experienced some degree of seasickness. (Bunting, 2016)

Producers of the popular TV show, *Deadliest Catch,* revealed that even Edgar Hansen of the *Northwestern* and Jonathan Hillstrand of *Time Bandit* still get seasick at the beginning of each season.

Who Gets Seasick (or Motion Sick)?

Seasickness and motion sickness can affect anyone. Ninety percent of all people suffer from some type of motion sickness during their lifetimes. Even experienced cruisers who have sailed dozens of times can get seasick. They don't stop cruising they just take precautions to lessen or prevent the seasickness. (Crislip, 2019)

Seasickness is especially bad when no one else seems to be afflicted, and it certainly is not limited to beginners. Knowing that about half the astronauts take motion sickness medication when in space should make you feel a little better.

People who are prone to motion sickness in cars, airplanes, or carnival rides may also be more susceptible to seasickness. However, the motion on different ships affects people differently. Just because you get seasick in a small boat does not mean you will have problems on a large cruise ship.

(Garrison, 2019)

Motion sickness is common and normal. Nearly anyone can be made motion sick by an appropriate stimulus. According to Benson, nearly 100% of (human) occupants of life rafts will vomit in rough seas and 60% of student aircrew members suffer from air sickness at some time during their training. About 7% of seagoing passengers report vomiting during a journey. (A. Lawther, 1988)

Horses, cows, monkeys, chimpanzees, birds and sheep have been reported in scientific publications to show motion sickness. Rats do not vomit so they cannot serve as experimental subjects.

Women are more sensitive to motion than men, by a ratio of about 5:3, although this may be related to reporting differences rather than true physiological differences. (Bob Cheung, 2001)

Women are more sensitive to motion around the times of their menstrual cycle. This may be due to interactions between migraine and motion sickness. (Grunfeld, 1999)

It has been reported that women of childbearing age become more prone to motion sickness as their migraine tendency increases. There are two spikes of migraine in women of childbearing age—one at 35, and another around menopause.

There are certain illnesses that eliminate motion sickness. These include bilateral loss of inner ear function (according to William James, the American

Pragmatist philospher), and lesions of the cerebellar nodulus (Bard). These illnesses are even worse than motion sickness, and there has been no attempt to use this observation clinically. (Timothy C. Hain, 2019)

According to studies, acquired susceptibility to motion sickness is rare.

People with rare, central nervous system disorders of the part of the brain that processes signals from the inner ear may also be unusually susceptible to motion sickness. Generally speaking, these are lesions of the cerebellum roof nuclei.

People with inner ear disturbance, especially a recent one, may be intolerant to activity in general. Certain individuals who are constitutionally susceptible to motion sickness, mainly women in mid-life, can develop seasickness on ships, and a prolonged land sickness, when they get off the ship. This rare disorder is called "mal de debarquement," which is French for "bad getting off the ship."

People with unusually good vestibular function may be more susceptible to motion sickness than others. (al, 1996)

People who have changes in their visual function—new glasses, laser eye surgery, progressive lenses, bifocals or trifocals, progressive contacts, mismatches between the size of images in one or the other ear, ocular misalignment—may develop more sensitivity to visual stimuli.

Research shows that people who are exposed to unusual visual environments, such as traders with nine different monitors, or air traffic controllers, may develop symptoms related to extreme amounts of visual stimulation. (Timothy C. Hain, 2019)

TIPS FROM CHAPTER 2

- Understand the history of seasickness and know that it happens to the best of us. At least you can know that you are in good company. Some of the world's greatest sailors and seamen have experienced seasickness.
- If you have recently had changes in your eyesight (new glasses, lasik surgery, new contact prescription, etc), you may be more susceptible to seasickness.
- If you are a migraine sufferer, you may be prone to seasickness and might wish to avoid any situation in which extreme motion occurs.
- If you are a woman, take precautions as research shows you may be more susceptible to seasickness and motion sickness than men.

CHAPTER 3

How to Prevent Seasickness

It's often been said that the only way to prevent seasickness is to sit under an apple tree. This makes perfect sense because there are obviously no apple trees at sea. It also implies that unless you are on land sitting under an apple tree, you will most likely get seasick at some point in your life.

I've talked to so many sailors who say, "I've never been seasick...well, except for this one time when ..." I'll say it again, there are two kinds of sailors. Those who get seasick, and those who lie about it.

According to medical experts, you can't catch seasickness. It is not a virus, although sometimes if people around you are sick, it makes you feel that way, too. There are three main seasickness triggers that should be avoided during your first few hours at sea.

1. Do not go below deck for extended time periods. Try to find a window or porthole and keep your eyes gazing (but not fixed) on the horizon.
2. Do not look through binoculars for long periods of time.
3. Do not stare at objects your brain will interpret as stable. Anything that involves staring at one point such as reading a book, doing detailed needlework, staring at screens, or even staring at a compass might bring on a bout of seasickness. (Garrison, 2019)

In addition to Garrison's three triggers, I'll add my own point of view of what can help to avoid seasickness—or at least quell its effects. For me and many other sailors, these are the five primary triggers for seasickness.

1. Fear
2. Food
3. Fatigue
4. Temperature
5. Hydration

For me, fear is the key trigger because I also believe that seasickness is psychological. It's really difficult to overcome fear, but I can recommend trying to stay as calm as possible to help avoid the horrible effects of seasickness. This is easier said than done, I realize. I also believe that experience helps with fear. And for a sailor, the only way to truly get experience and the confidence that comes with it is to get out there and sail. The fear and anxiety, in my opinion, contributes significantly to the possibility of seasickness.

Food is also important. If you have an empty stomach, or if you eat the wrong kinds of food (like spicy, fatty, or acidic food), your tummy may not cooperate in a pleasant way when the nausea sets in. As you will read in future chapters, I've also learned to eat food items before a long passage based on the "reverse taste." For example, a banana or an apple tastes a lot better coming back up than tuna or yogurt. Trust me, I've learned this the hard way!

Fatigue can also contribute to the potential of seasickness. It's always a good idea to be well rested before setting sail, especially if the weather is questionable or if it's a long offshore passage. Seasickness itself can make you drowsy, and most seasickness medications will most certainly make you sleepy, so try and be well rested before departure.

Temperature, I believe, is also a key factor. I tend to get more nauseous when it's extremely cold or extremely hot. Try to dress appropriately for the weather and be prepared for temperature changes.

And finally, hydration is key. Stay well hydrated the day before and the morning of departure. This means staying away from alcohol, too! Also, even if you continue to throw it right back up, try to stay hydrated during bouts with seasickness. Even a few drops of water can help to quell the nausea. Also, if you are like me and continue to vomit even when there is nothing left in your tummy, the heaving will be less horrible if there is at least a little liquid in your belly to dilute the harsh taste and vile smell of stomach acid.

Staying busy and keeping your mind occupied are also great ways to avoid seasickness. Try to stay on deck in the fresh air and focus on anything other than the moving ship. Take deep breaths and drink plenty of water. When on deck, facing forward (rather than to the side) seems to help most people. Remember that you need to let your brain adjust to this new unstable environment by allowing the horizon to act as the true point of reference.

If you are on a cruise ship, try lying down in a deck chair in the fresh air and try to sleep it off. Most modern cruise ships are equipped with stabilizers that eliminate much of the motion that causes seasickness. This is one time when bigger might be better—the larger the ship, the less it will rock. If you know you are prone to seasickness, try to get a cabin on the outside (with a window), and mid-ship and on a lower deck where there is less motion.

Cruising in relatively calm waters may also help those prone to seasickness. The Caribbean (except during hurricane season) is usually calm, as is the Inside Passage to Alaska. River cruises are also a good choice. (Garrison, 2019)

But my experience is on small sailboats, not large cruise ships. I do think these tips are great advice, but some of them may not work for small-vessel sailors and small crews when sometimes you can't sleep because you must cover your shift.

TIPS FROM CHAPTER 3

- Do not go below deck for extended time periods.
- Try to find a window or porthole and keep your eyes gazing (but not fixed) on the horizon.
- Do not look through binoculars for long periods of time.
- Do not stare at objects your brain will interpret as stable. Anything that involves staring at one point such as reading a book, doing detailed

needlework, or even staring at a compass might bring on a bout of seasickness.

- Try to relax and not focus on your fears. The anxiety of fear can greatly contribute to seasickness.
- Keep something on your belly and consider the reverse tastes of food (for example, an apple or banana tastes a lot better coming back up that tuna or yogurt).
- Try to keep a stable temperature and dress appropriately for the weather. Extreme cold and extreme heat can contribute to seasickness.
- Stay hydrated! Hydrate well the day before and the morning of departure. This means avoiding alcohol and also taking a few sips of water, even during heavy bouts of vomiting.
- Staying busy and keeping your mind occupied are the best ways to avoid seasickness.
- Try to stay on deck in the fresh air and focus on anything other than the moving ship.
- Take deep breaths and drink plenty of water.
- When on deck, facing forward (rather than to the side) seems to help most people.
- Remember that you need to let your brain adjust to this new unstable environment by allowing the horizon to act as the true point of reference.
- Try to eat, but avoid spicy, acidic, or fatty food.

- If possible, cruise in relatively calm waters.

CHAPTER 4

Facing Fear and Seasickness in The Baltic Sea

Fear is one of the most dangerous psychological factors that can contribute to seasickness. I learned this the hard way when we set sail on our worldwide voyage on August 19, 2018 from Stralsund, Germany.

With only the one seasickness experience (from Rønne, Denmark to Karliskrona, Sweden in May 2016) under my belt, I didn't expect a repeat of the debilitating effects of motion sickness. Fear was most certainly a factor. Here are the grueling details as we set sail to Battle the Baltic.

Battling the Baltic (Part One)

Anticipation had grown as the excitement began to swell in sync with the Baltic Sea waves. We were already 18 days past our original departure date, but we wanted to be absolutely certain that the ship and the crew were ready! After five years of talking about this and almost a year of intense planning, we finally made the decision that on Sunday, August 19, 2018, at 09:00 we would set sail on the first leg of our sailing voyage that will take us across the Atlantic from Stralsund, Germany to Plash Island in Gulf Shores, Alabama.

We checked off our final list and frantically took care of the final details. Thilo, our superb electrician and mechanic, wrapped up his final tasks and cleared the electrical systems ready to set sail. We made one last provision run, and I washed some clothes and gave our canine crew—beagles Cap'n Jack and Scout—a bath. I secured all the items in the cabin that could be tossed and thrown during rough conditions.

We turned the boat's bow toward the bridge to the entertaining delight of a very large crowd dining in the outdoor restaurant right next to our mooring.

We finished getting everything ready and took a proper shower. With no shower on board our ship, *Seefalke*, we needed to walk a mile to the machine shop to use the mechanics' shower. It was greasy and oily, but the water was hot. I FaceTimed with my children, Shelby and Bo, and then we took the dogs on a long walk and had a nice dinner. We knew we needed rest, but the excitement and anticipation kept us from relaxing. We set the alarm for 06:00 and forced ourselves to sleep.

First Stop—Sailing to Kiel, Germany (approx. 100 nm)
SUNDAY, 19 AUGUST 2018
Stralsund, Germany—Departure Time 09:00

The skipper bounced out of bed at 05:30, long before any alarm sounded. I tried to squeeze in the last 30 minutes of sleep, but my brain would not stop swirling, so I decided it might be best if I bounce out of bed too.

I took care of feeding and walking the dogs and securing the cabins, while we got the boat ready. I continued to fight the battle between nerves and excitement. It's hard to say which one was winning. They were both taking their punches.

It was just minutes before 09:00 and our celebration flags were flying high. The Seadogs were securely tethered, and the weather was clear and beautiful. We toasted the journey and gave Neptune a shot of whiskey to ensure a safe voyage.

The bridge began to open, and we thrusted into line and went happily through the bridge and into the Baltic Sea—waters we know very well. We put up two of the sails and were cruising along nicely for about four hours.

With no warning, the waves began to roll and swell to about two meters high. We began to fight against the currents and the wind. We safely secured Cap'n Jack and Scout in the cabin below and took our seasickness medicine. In hindsight, we should have taken it earlier.

We were pushing heavily against the wind and the current was attacking us—pushing us back further than we could move forward. It was a battle of nature against man and ship. And while *Seefalke* was holding her own, nature seemed to be beating the humans by a landslide.

It's in moments like these that you forget how soothing the sea can be and you remember its power and force.

We continuously adjusted the sails, switching back and forth from the genoa and a smaller jib. We reefed the main and continued to tack and fight and battle the Baltic, which clearly did not want us invading her home on this day.

I began to feel queasy and told myself to fight it.

Look at the horizon. Ignore the motion that is slamming us. Stay busy. Think of something else.

I worked hard to convince my brain that I didn't feel the harsh effects of the roller coaster that was once the Baltic. The harder I tried to convince myself I wasn't getting seasick, the more the uneasy feeling took over.

I looked at the skipper and told him I was about to lose it. Within 15 seconds of that statement, I leaned over the port side deck outside the cockpit and spewed all the cereal and yogurt from the morning's breakfast onto the stern.

At first, I felt ok after emptying my belly. *I have been seasick before and this was not as bad as that last time. I just fed a few fish. I'm really ok.*

But as the ship continued to sway back and forth, and up and down, my body finally gave in and let the Baltic win the battle. I got comfortable in my position over the side of the boat, strapped myself in, and stayed there for a couple of hours.

It didn't take long for my belly to empty completely, but the contractions and heaving continued until I was literally throwing up only stomach acid and possibly pieces of my stomach lining. It was so forceful, I actually peed in my pants uncontrollably. I was embarrassed, but at the same time I really didn't care.

I worked my way into the cabin below to find some clean panties. This is when I realized I had done a terrible job of securing the cabin items. Almost all of the cabin's contents were in heaps and piles of disorganized rubble. It looked like someone had shaken the boat like a cup of dice and thrown its contents into the belly of the boat. I somehow made it through the messy maze to the head and cleaned myself, but then realized I needed to get comfortable again and just hug the toilet for a while.

I lay on the floor, lifeless, for about another hour, completely paralyzed and unable to get up from that spot. Seriously, if someone held a gun to my head and told me to move one inch, I would have just had to let them pull the trigger. I could not move.

At one point, I looked at the puppies, sitting so sweetly in their little bed in the cabin saloon, all cuddled up and being so good. I could tell they were worried about me, but fortunately, they seemed fine.

I grabbed a trash bag to hopefully catch anything else that might want to exit my body and worked my way to the table bench in the saloon and just crashed. I kept apologizing to the skipper, and he kept reassuring me. The pressure of not pulling my own weight was making it worse. It was adding anxiety to the mix of nerves and excitement. I wanted to help him. But I couldn't.

After 12 hours, the waters began to calm, and we decided to anchor for the night. As soon as the motion stopped, so did my misery. This is the amazing thing about this phenomenon we call seasickness. When the motion ends, the sickness ends. I got up and felt just fine cruising along on the calm waters. I helped him drop and secure the anchor and then walked the pups on the deck. We had sailed for 12 hours in these brutal conditions. By the time we got the ship secure, it was around 23:00 and we all went immediately to sleep.

Trouble at Anchor - Anchored near Prerow Shoal, just North of Darsser Or
MONDAY, 20 AUGUST 2018

At 03:30, the skipper bolted out of bed. "The anchor is dragging," he said. He is an experienced sailor and can *feel* things that others can only see or hear. I sprang to my feet, too, and we both leaped onto the deck in our skivvies.

The water was no longer calm. Two-meter waves were rolling us and providing a cold saltwater shower as they crashed onto the bow. The heavy wind was chapping our faces and pushing all of *Seefalke's* 11 tons. We turned on the engine and tried to retrieve the anchor, but the chain got jumbled inside the windlass and completely jammed it. It wouldn't drop down and it couldn't be retrieved. The anchor was dangling from the bow sprit, and we feared it would strike *Seefalke* and rip into her bow. We tried manually to retrieve the anchor, but it wouldn't budge.

We fought and tugged with all our might. Finally, we were able to attach a line and leverage our weight to pull up the anchor and secure it. It was now 03:45 and we had no choice but to move forward. We didn't even try to put up a sail. We cranked the motor and forged ahead. We both took more seasickness medicine.

It was pitch black dark.

Battling Seasickness and the Baltic

For some reason, when you can't see the motion, your body tells you it's not there, even though you can feel it. At least this seems to be how it was for me at this time. I've read a lot about seasickness. It is an interesting phenomenon and has a lot to do with balance of the inner ear, the sinuses, blood flow, heart rhythm, hydration, and many psychological factors including nerves, excitement, and fear. Different parts of your body send different signals to your brain. The wires get tangled and the confusion of all these crossed signals to the brain can cause the uneasiness.

As the sun began to rise, so did the empty insides of my belly. The skipper told me to go down below and sleep for two hours. I did. The entire time the boat was rocking, but I felt ok. I returned to relieve the skipper, and he said he would try to sleep for two hours. So, I took my shift. But I basically just strapped myself in the cockpit and held on for dear life for 120 straight minutes.

The skipper returned two hours later, as promised, and I went below to rest another two hours. This is where I made a crucial mistake. I should have stayed in the fresh air where I felt fine and steady. I lay down on the bunk and felt it all set in again. I could feel something rising in my throat and ran to the head as fast as I could...just in time. Then I hugged the toilet for the next couple hours. There was zero food in my belly, so I'm not sure what was still coming up. But something was. At one point, the skipper checked on me because he saw my lifeless body sprawled out on the floor and thought I was passed out.

If you've never been seasick, let me try to describe it for you.

Imagine the worst hangover you've ever had, combined with the worst possible food poisoning. Then throw in a nasty case of Type A flu complete with vomiting, chills, cold sweat, and a pounding, throbbing headache. Then, feeling all of this simultaneously, put yourself inside a washing machine and turn it on the fast spin cycle. Then, just to get the full effect, hop onto the fastest, most swirly, most topsy-turvy roller coaster you can find. This is kind of what it feels like. Complete disorientation. Boiling vile in your stomach and throat ripping through your innards and tossing and turning your insides out. Gut-wrenching heaving that you can feel in every part of your body. It literally jerks your body from your waist as if it were attached to a hook on a crane.

Then imagine all your muscles starting to cramp as the dehydration paralyzes you. Some people see visions, and others just completely black out. I can remember sailing from Rönne, Denmark to Karlskrona, Sweden a few years ago. That was the worst seasickness I've ever experienced. The captain had to D-ring strap me to the boat to keep me from falling out...or from throwing myself out, because that is what I wanted to do. This was not as bad as that, which is the only positive thing I can say about it. I guess I also wanted to lose some weight, but I will never recommend the Nordic Seafarer's Diet to anyone!

And all this doesn't stop until the motion stops. Curiously, when the motion does finally stop, you feel just fine. When I'm not experiencing seasickness, I'm fascinated by it.

We rolled into Rostock around 16:00 and just as soon as we were on calm waters, I felt just fine. Absolutely fine. I was able to jump up, get on the deck, secure the mooring lines, secure the fenders, and help to moor *Seefalke*. After six hours of utter and complete misery, I felt just fine.

I took the dogs on a long walk and cooked dinner. I even cleaned the entire boat and re-organized all the items that had scattered all over the cabins. We went to bed early and got some much-needed sleep.

Assessing the Damage from Brutal Sailing Conditions
TUESDAY, 21 AUGUST 2018 —Hohe-Düne Marina

We got some sleep and awoke to assess the damage. It was severe. We knew the anchor windlass was broken. But we didn't know that all the bolted down boards of the bow sprit had been blown away. There was nothing there. Nothing. We also realized that one of the sheets of the genoa had gotten tangled underneath *Seefalke* and chewed up inside the motor of the bow thruster. This reminds me of when you roll your vacuum cleaner over a cord and the cord just gets sucked up into the mechanism and cannot be retrieved.

The skipper tore apart the cabins that I had so carefully organized, again, and began to work on the repairs. He discovered that the anchor windlass just needed a new fuse, but he had to completely empty the bow cabin to get to it. He then knew that he would have to take a swim underneath *Seefalke* to try and untangle the line that was sucked into the bow thruster. We measured the space on the bow sprit where three heavy boards were bolted down tightly just one day before. They were gone. The Baltic apparently ate them for dinner—a nice entrée after the appetizer of my belly contents.

I set out on a hunt for supplies. Hohe-Düne is a gorgeous marina, however, it's a bit fancy and "high society" for our taste. I think this is where huge yacht owners moor their vessels and leave them for someone else to repair while they go stay in a five-star hotel. There were no marine shops to be found. I took a ferry into Warnemunde and searched for supplies there. No luck. After about four hours, I returned to *Seefalke* empty handed. A failed mission. Again, I felt the disappointment of not being at all helpful for my captain.

The skipper decided to swim under the boat and was able to disengage the mangled line from the bow thruster. He had to cut the line to get it out, so this added another sheet to the list of supplies that I had already failed to find. But the good news is that we only had to replace the line and not the bow thruster. It was now working just fine.

We decided to go into Rostock to look for the fuse and boards. We took the ferry back into Warnemunde then took a train into Rostock. The pups were loving all the new smells as they always do when we stop at these different ports. We walked two kilometers to the marine shop. They didn't have the boards we needed or the correct fuse voltage, but we found a fuse that would work.

When we returned to *Seefalke*, the skipper was able to quickly fix the anchor windlass and then I spent the next two hours putting everything back into its proper compartments and securing all our belongings....AGAIN. I logged more than 28,000 steps on my FitBit that day.

We showered in the marina facilities and went to bed early looking forward to another day of rest. I planned to do laundry the next day and catch up on some work. But the Baltic had something different in mind.

Fair Winds and Following Seas on the Baltic
WEDNESDAY, 22 AUGUST 2018—Departure for Heiligenhafen (Grossenbrode, Germany)

There is a popular saying for those who sail regularly on the Baltic Sea. "If you don't like the weather, wait an hour."

The weather here changes on a dime. I can remember sailing on the Baltic one afternoon when our port side was sunny and calm with blue skies that reminded me of a warm sunny day in Alabama. To the starboard side, the skies were black with high waves swelling and coming toward us—complete with thunder and heavy rain. It was that different to the right and to the left of us.

We awoke in Hohe-Düne to a gorgeous sunrise, calm waters, and favorable winds. The skipper went to the washroom to shave and made a decision that would instantly change our well-planned day of rest. He texted me that we needed to take advantage of the conditions, get the boat ready, and set sail around 10:00. I got the pups fed and walked then decided to unleash the hounds and let them play on the beach for about half an hour so they would be a bit worn out for whatever the Baltic had in mind for us today.

We got the boat ready and I carefully collected seasickness medicine, crackers, water, bananas, ginger tea, and any other supplies I could think of that we could put in a handy place in the cockpit—just in case. This time, I would be prepared.

As bitter as the Baltic had been on our first two days at sea, on this day she was as sweet as pumpkin pie!

Under a perfectly sunny, bright blue sky, we sailed at about 3.5 knots along the sea that was now welcoming us into her nurturing arms. It was so calm we were able to do a little work, and I took the first shift at the helm. We put up four sails and were even able to play with the Drone a little and get some remarkable photos and video of *Seefalke* under sail on a perfect afternoon.

We sailed 43.4 nautical miles in 14 hours into Großenbrode. It was midnight when we began to get close to the Heiligenhafen Marina. We had never been in this marina and it was pitch black, so we decided to anchor for the night right outside the marina.

Oh, how we needed this day to simply enjoy the sailing, relax, and NOT be seasick! This reminded me why we do this.

Boat Repairs and Boat Maintenance
THURSDAY, 23 AUGUST 2018—
Heiligenhafen (Grossenbrode, Germany)

A day of rest and recovery and real work was needed. We both got a lot accomplished and as a bonus, I got to connect with my lifelong friend, Yvonne Habermann.

Yvi, a native of Hamburg, lived with our family in Decatur, Alabama when she was an exchange student in the late 1980s. The first time I ever went sailing was with Yvi in Hamburg in 2013.

Many years ago, Yvi took two long voyages in a very small, 7-meter sailboat that took her along the same path that we are taking. She didn't cross the Atlantic, but she covered much of the same waters along the Baltic, the North Sea, and around the European Atlantic coast and into Morocco. She gave me great advice and a lot of confidence that I can do it, too.

We talked a lot about seasickness and how to fight it. She recommended either standing up or lying flat when the sickness sets in. She also said one of the best things to do is simply stay busy and perhaps even stand up and take the wheel. This will help to focus on the horizon and also gives you a sense of control of the motion, she said. Great advice from an awesome girl sailor who totally rocks!

She confirmed the notion that seasickness can be psychological. She told me that years ago when she was a sailing instructor, she would tell students that if they just held a potato in their left hand, then they wouldn't get seasick. This mind over matter worked for most of them. I have some potatoes on board, and I'm willing to try anything.

We got ready to make the final move toward Kiel the next morning. We estimated it was around 30 nautical miles, but we could face heavy currents the second half of the day and will definitely face cold and rain—perhaps even thunderstorms.

Battling the Baltic Part Two
Friday, 24 August 2018

The Baltic Sea is a bitch.

She's like the queen of the mean girls in high school. You know the one ... the girl who is beautiful and talented, engaging and alluring. She's the girl who every boy wants to date and who every other girl wants to be. Everyone loves her, and everyone hates her.

When she's nice, she can make you feel like the most important and wonderful human on the planet. But rub her the wrong way or catch her in a bad mood, and there will be pure Hell to pay! You won't see it coming. It will blindside you and leave you scratching your head wondering what you did to piss her off.

Make no mistake—I am in love with the Baltic. I learned to sail on the Baltic and have been sailing on her since 2013. The Baltic Sea is gorgeous. She is alluring and engaging, and I thought I was her friend. I'm not sure why she is turning on me this week.

Let me make one thing clear. I am the girl who doesn't care if the mean girl likes me or not. I generally just admire her from afar and find other friends in other circles. I'm not interested in the drama. But I'm also the girl who will not get beaten up or beaten down without a fight. I'm just not that girl. At least that's been my heartfelt belief for the past 51 years.

During our first week on this cross-Atlantic voyage, the Baltic forced me to question that belief. This mean girl has gotten the best of me. I spent two days of utter misery over the side of our sailing vessel, *Seefalke,* fighting a mean girl that just didn't want me on her turf. She had mercy on me one day and reminded me why I love her so much. But was this just her way of manipulating me to come back for more?

During this journey, we had only one more day on the Baltic. I was determined to defeat the mean girl who was torturing me.

It was a rainy and windy morning when we left Heiligenhafen. We knew that the weather report called for heavy winds and currents against us... again. And it was cold. But we decided to forge ahead anyway.

I was nervous and afraid. I wasn't afraid of the weather or the conditions or the sailing. My fear was with fighting the seasickness again. At least there would be no surprises this time because we knew the weather would be rough. I gave myself a pep talk and tried to stay busy with preparations. I told myself that I wouldn't let The Baltic Sea beat me down again. She had rewarded our early week battles with a gorgeous day of slow, relaxed cruising. But who knew what kind of mood she would be in on this cold, wet day.

We had three options. First, a straight route directly to Kiel. But there was a military exercise zone right in the middle of our route, so we needed to continue to listen to the radio to avoid this. There was a chance we would hit that pocket at the end of the exercise and could push through. Second option was to re-route just a little to avoid the artillery. Or, third, we could swing around it entirely, which would add five hours to the passage and provide an even tougher battle with the currents.

After feeding and walking our four-legged crew, Cap'n Jack and Scout, I bundled into my cold weather gear and helped get *Seefalke* ready. Staying busy was keeping my mind off my fear of another day of over-the-rail puking.

We got out to sea with the rain and wind, but it was not bad at all—at first. We got the pups settled down below and got the smaller jib and main sail hoisted. We had double-reefed the main ahead of time in preparation for the inevitable heavy wind.

We had chosen not to drink coffee that morning in preparation of avoiding anything acidic or lactic in our bellies. I was fighting to keep my eyes open, so I decided to take a short nap. This would also help to relax me, I hoped. The puppies hopped onto the bunk next to me for some extra cuddles, and I let them.

Probably an hour or so later I awoke to a rocking boat. I could hear the skipper rushing around on the deck above and caught glimpses through the upper hatch windows of him adjusting the sails. The boat began to tilt and a few of my well-secured items went flying across the cabin. *Damn! Am I ever going to get that stupid puzzle to fit together correctly?*

Then the pups and I both began to slide. I didn't know it at the time, but we were in the middle of a heavy gale-force thunderstorm with winds at 38 knots! We were on a 36-degree tilt ... and by the way, the skipper was having the time of his life.

I was laying flat on my back on the bunk. My right leg was stretched out straight and propped against the board that generally keeps the pups secure in their bed. My left leg was bent and upright, blocking the pups from flying across the cabin with the various items that were still not secured. I couldn't move to secure the pups in their bunk. I could only hold on to keep them safe as we were practically vertical at this point. They were barely fazed at all, but I was using every muscle in my body to stabilize myself, and them, in this awkward position.

I think this is what yoga is supposed to feel like— holding one unusual, uncomfortable position as long as possible while your muscles flex and spasm.

I called up to the cockpit to be sure I wasn't needed. The skipper looked down at me and had the biggest, silliest grin on his face. I thought to myself, *"What are you smiling about?"* He was loving the challenge of fighting the storm. "Just keep holding on," he said.

Then an alarm sounded.

It was coming from the bilge and this meant water had gotten in and risen to a level that would trip the alarm. The skipper told me to check it out. *What? Are you kidding me? How the hell will I get out of this position without slamming into the other side of the cabin?*

First, I had to secure the pups. I somehow got them settled and surrounded them with three sleeping bags to give them extra padding. They were now in their usual barricaded bed, which stabilizes them in a confined space and keeps them from moving around in the boat. They curled up and went right back to sleep. *Why can't I be that relaxed?*

Then I needed to get to the bilge, which meant pulling up the floor covering and opening the two hatches that led down below to *Seefalke's* stomach. I was doing all this on a 36-degree tilt during gale-force winds. I felt like I was in one of those old black-and-white movies where the room spins, and the actors dance around on the walls and the ceiling.

There was a little water in *Seefalke's* belly, but not enough for concern. I closed the hatches and plopped back down on the bed, this time with both legs giving me leverage.

It was a forceful squall, but a short one. Soon, we were back on some sort of evenness, and I could see through the upper hatch window that the skipper had pulled in the jib. It was flapping just a little on the edge. I asked if everything was ok, and he again looked down with a ridiculously happy grin . . . so I knew I was ok to just stay put. He was fine.

How a Sailor Battles a Storm and the Fear Within

I wanted to go back to the cockpit. But I was afraid.

In fact, I was paralyzed.

Paralyzed with fear.

Again, there was no fear of the boat or the conditions. I was afraid that if I got up, I would hurl and spend the rest of the day in misery. I didn't feel sick or queasy at all, but the fear of getting sick again was keeping me from going back to the cockpit.

I lay there for what seemed like hours, just staring blankly through the hatch window at the flapping jib. I don't even think I blinked. I was hypnotized. I don't know why. I learned to sail on the Baltic. I had spent the past five years sailing on the Baltic. I love The Baltic Sea! She's my friend. *Why was she kicking my ass this time?*

I knew that this was the last time we would be sailing on her during this trip. Once we get to Kiel, we sail through the Kiel Canal and then meet the challenging North Sea on the other side. *I'm wasting my time down here when I should be up there sailing the Baltic!*

I remembered a wise old saying. "The brave one is not the one who has no fear. The brave one is the one who has fear . . . but does it anyway."

Then I just snapped out of it.

I got up and said to myself, *"If I get sick, I get sick. I need to be out there."*

How a Sailor Overcomes Fear

The boat was still rocking, but it was manageable. I could see the high waves through the portholes. I put on my life vest and walked up the four stairs to the cockpit. The skipper was standing on the cockpit bench, wind in his face, wearing the biggest smile I've ever seen. *How could I possibly be afraid of this?* I have a captain who lives for this shit!

He is not going to let anything happen to us. He is happy and in his element—facing the sea and the storm with absolute joy! I stood up on the bench, too, and let the cold wind chill my face and blow my hair. It was exhilarating. I had wasted seven hours in the cabin below fearing something that usually makes me so happy. And in this moment, I remembered why.

We can battle the sea, or we can embrace it. Sometimes she will be sweet, and sometimes mean as a snake. But either way, this is her turf. We must embrace the experience and trust that we will get through it. *If I get sick, I get sick.* But I'm out here, and I have this opportunity to challenge myself. I may not beat the Baltic, and I can't expect to... but I will NOT beat myself!

We still had four hours to Kiel, and the Baltic was breathtaking. *Seefalke* was surfing on the two-meter waves like she was performing a choreographed dance to a mesmerized and appreciative audience. We were all flying.

Yes, the Baltic Sea is a bitch. She can be bitter one day and sugary-sweet the next. But I love her.

TIPS FROM CHAPTER 4

- Nerves, excitement, and fear can contribute to seasickness. Try to stay calm the day of departure.
- Try to get a good night's sleep the night before departure.
- Take a good shower before departure so you feel refreshed.

48

- Eat well the night before departure.
- Avoid alcohol the night before departure and during the passage.
- If you choose to take seasickness medicine, it's best to take it about two hours before departure. Once the seasickness sets in, it's too late.
- Try to avoid medicine that will make you drowsy if you know you have a shift at the helm within 6 hours.
- When you begin to feel queasy, stay busy. Grab the wheel, to feel a sense of control, or focus on a small task.
- When conditions get rough, reef the main sail and adjust the sails in a way that cushions the motion.
- Stay in the fresh air, if possible.
- Try not to focus on the queasiness. Find anything else to focus on!
- Lie flat in the center part of the ship with your eyes closed. Try to sleep, if possible.
- Rest when you can, even if you don't feel tired.
- Either stand up or lie flat on your back when you feel the seasickness set in. Don't sit.
- Hold a potato in your left hand. Sometimes mind over matter works if you truly believe it.
- Try not to let fear paralyze you.
- Don't feel bad about succumbing to the seasickness and trust the rest of the crew will help you. This kind of anxiety can make the seasickness worse.
- Trust your captain to alleviate the fear that you may be in danger.

- Trust your ship to get you to your destination safely.
- Trust yourself and try to reassure yourself that everything will be Ok.
- Remember: "The brave one is not the one who has no fear. The brave one is the one who has fear... but does it anyway."
- Embrace the things you love about being on the water and try to focus on the good things rather than the queasiness or the fear.

CHAPTER 5

Finding Sea Legs in the English Channel

A 20-degree angle may not seem like much at first glance. If you look at it on an axis it's barely even an incline. However, if you are on a sailboat flying through the water at a 20-degree tilt for, let's say, four or five straight days and nights, and you are trying to perform daily living activities . . . well, then it may as well be a 90-degree angle.

You are just sideways. All the time.

If you've never been on a sailboat, try to imagine walking on a steep hill—but you are not walking forward. You are walking sideways. Now imagine that the hill is moving. It's rocking back and forth at times. Sometimes, the slant increases and sometimes it decreases. The speed changes constantly.

And oh, by the way . . . there are also 10-to-15-knot winds blowing at you from another direction. Now, try to think about walking along sideways on this slanting, moving hill and also trying to cook dinner, or eat dinner, or brush your teeth, or pee in the potty without missing. Everything you do—even just standing or sleeping—requires balancing your entire body and holding on with at least one hand.

I should have good balance. In my youth I competed in gymnastics. I did flips and twists and leaps on a balance beam—a four-inch piece of wood positioned four feet off the ground.

That was hard.

It's possible this is harder.

At least the balance beam wasn't moving, and each routine lasted only 90 seconds.

When you live on a moving sailboat, even when you are sleeping you are holding on. You must position yourself on the bunk so that you don't slide right off into the floor. Or worse, you hold on to avoid getting thrown against the other side of the cabin. And just as you get to a point where you feel some sense of balance, the wind shifts, and you must tack. This means changing direction by shifting the sails to the other side. Then the boat tilts the other way, and you have to re-balance yourself on the opposite side.

You train yourself to find balance. You learn to hold on. You learn to perform regular, daily tasks one-handed. You bend your knees and perform a slow-motion, hula-hoop action with the lower part of your body to cushion and balance the movement.

This is pretty much what it was like for 92 straight hours as we sailed 348 nautical miles in five days, nonstop, through The English Channel from St.-Valéry-en-Caux, France to Camaret-sur-Mer, France. We crossed into the open North Atlantic Ocean and now wait on weather good enough to face our greatest challenge yet—The Bay of Biscay.

But more about that later. I don't want to overshadow the accomplishment and challenge of the voyage through The English Channel. You can read the full English Channel story on my blog, but here is a condensed recap...

   While in port, we stayed busy working on strategically planning each leg of our voyage. It generally takes about two to three hours creating each of our passage plans. We carefully study several different weather sources, and pour through the Reed's Nautical Almanac and all the paper charts required for each voyage. Then we try to determine just the right time for departure to best take advantage of the weather, wind, currents, and conditions. Then we determined the best route.

   Due to the tides and the wind, we would spend the first part of the voyage with barely any wind and would motor sail slowly through The Channel for about a day and a half. Then the wind and currents would be against us, and we would have to fight some uncomfortable battles. We waited several days for more favorable conditions.

   During that time, I thought about a recent voyage—nonstop across the North Sea. I had made two critical mistakes during this passage. They were critical enough that I considered just giving up on this whole journey (read my blog "The Night Watch Video Game").

   Reliving it was brutal. I could barely talk about it without bursting into tears. I was feeling a lot of fear and anticipation of making mistakes again during the next passage. The captain kept telling me to quit worrying about it, but this was frustrating me even more. He perhaps just can't understand some of the emotions that I was going through.

This is a grand experience, and I'm grateful every single day for the opportunity to challenge myself. But I can't pretend that it's all just sailing and sunshine all the time. Most of the time I love it! I love the challenge and the adventure. But sometimes it's hard. Sometimes it's not fun. Sometimes it rips me to shreds from the inside out—probably because I'm still a novice and it just requires more effort for me.

For seasoned sailors, it's innate. It's so much a part of their soul that it just comes naturally. But I also try to remember that it's the hard parts that make it special. If it was easy, anyone could do it.

ENGLISH CHANNEL LEG 2 – DAY 1 AT SEA

The next morning, I was feeling a bit less emotional. It's amazing what a good night of sleep can do for you mentally. I took a long walk with the pups and went to the grocery store for fresh fruit and vegetables.

When we returned to the boat, I slipped on the concrete stairs walking down to the floating pier. They were slippery and slimy from the earlier high tide. When the tide goes down every six hours, there is a slimy film left on some of the lower stairs. I had been thinking all week that I might slip on them. And I finally did. I fell mostly on my bum, which is the most padded part of my body, but I also twisted my right foot forward trying to catch my fall and stubbed my big toe badly, ripping the entire nail from the flesh.

It's just a toe, but damn that hurt! How can something so small hurt so much? My shoe filled with blood. It was throbbing, but of course, I tried not to cry because the captain hates it when I cry. So, instead, I washed it off and bandaged it and said a few four-letter words that would embarrass my mother. And then I just moved on.

We spent the morning studying the weather and around 13:30 that afternoon we decided we needed to set sail at high tide, which would be around 15:00. We learned that the bridge would open at 15:30, so we frantically began preparations.

I was already not feeling well. My toe was throbbing, I was worried about my dad because he was having cataract surgery that morning. And now I felt rushed. We generally have more time to prepare for departure. Of course, even though it was chaotic, we got it done. But emotions and tensions were already high.

We departed at 15:30 as planned. The high water was producing huge waves as we left the marina and ventured back into The English Channel. I was still marveling at the gorgeous green color of the water—a color I still can't quite describe, but I know I will never forget it.

We were fighting the groundswells and the currents, but it was time to put up the sails. I hoisted the main, but not without some struggles. Then the captain said we needed to hoist the jib and asked me if I wanted to go to the bow to do it or hold the wheel and keep us in the wind. The currents were forceful and so was the wind, so I decided it was best if the captain kept *Seefalke* steady.

I crawled onto the bow.

The wind was howling and the boat was rocking in what seemed like all directions. We were already on at least a 20-degree tilt, so I had to position my body in just the right way to be able to stabilize myself with my legs while working with both hands to untie the jib ties. I got the first two loose, but there was a huge knot in the tie that was securing the jib boom. It took me several minutes to untangle the knot, although it seemed like forever. I finally got it loose and hoisted the jib as the boom swiftly flew over to the starboard side to join the main boom. I had to hang on with both arms and legs to keep from flying across the boat along with the sails.

I crawled back to the cockpit, feeling relatively proud of my accomplishment. I've hoisted the main and the jib a million times, but these were extremely rough conditions, so I was pleased with myself. Even the captain told me I did a good job, which he never does, so this made me so happy. I felt a bit queasy and uneasy from the extreme motion. Then I was instructed to hoist the mizzen. This is the sail located on the stern. This wasn't as difficult because the two other sails were cushioning the effects of the waves by this time.

I was feeling queasy, but was fighting the good fight. The captain handed me Yvi's potato. This made me laugh and relieved some of my tension and uneasiness. My friend Yvi was previously a sailing instructor and she told me she would tell her students to just hold a potato in their left hand to prevent seasickness. Sometimes mind over matter is the best cure. I held Yvi's potato in my left hand. It was working. I wanted to take the first shift since it was still daylight. I took the helm from 16:00 until 20:00, just before sunset.

It was a beautiful afternoon, but the wind was strong and we were already on that 20-degree tilt. I was battling the queasiness and the ever-challenging balancing act had already begun. But I tried to focus on the beauty that surrounded me. As the sun was setting, it was reflecting on the gorgeous green water. It looked like the sea was filled with sparkling diamonds. As my shift came to an end, I wondered if I would ever see that green color again.

Battling Nerves and Seasickness During a Challenging Sailing Passage
Wednesday, 12 September 2018
SAILING THE ENGLISH CHANNEL LEG 2 - DAY 2 AT SEA

I awakened at 02:00 for my night shift to discover that we were fighting against the currents. The wind was coming from one direction, but the currents were moving in a different direction—against us. This was causing the waves to be confused and rocky, and the currents were pushing us backward.

I didn't sleep well, but I got myself mentally ready for my watch. It was a frustrating watch because we had to tack off course a little to wait on the wind the shift. So, I was basically backtracking right back over the course that the captain had taken earlier in the night. It was kind of a north-to-south reverse move. It was frustrating to feel like we weren't getting anywhere.

The night was black and foggy. There was not much traffic, which helped my nerves, but it was difficult to see anything. I got through the four-hour shift.

I needed to relax, but for some reason I just couldn't. I woke up a few hours later and was queasy and uneasy and just couldn't make myself get out of bed. I just lay there cuddling with Cap'n Jack and Scout for a couple hours. I finally came up to the cockpit around noon, but I just felt wretched. I tried to get my body and mind balanced, but it just wasn't working.

Around 12:30, I could feel the contents of my belly rising to my throat. I reached for the potato, but it was too late. I surrendered and made a sacrifice to the seasickness gods. I puked over the starboard side of *Seefalke*. This time, there was not much in my belly. We had not eaten a proper meal since the night before our departure, so it was mostly stomach acid—which is just about the most horrible thing you could ever taste.

This was the first time I had been seasick since our first two days at sea on The Baltic almost three weeks ago. I think we were at port for so long, perhaps I just lost my sea legs again. I was pissed at myself, even though I know it's not my fault. And I could see the captain's look of disappointment, as if he was wondering if I would be any help from this point on. In hindsight, I think it was actually a look of empathy. But

I couldn't help but feel once again that I wasn't going to be able to make any contribution.

I decided that this time I was not going to let seasickness control me for the next however many days we would be at sea in these rocky conditions.

I was still a bit unsteady and reached for a banana. I wanted to put something on my tummy that didn't taste like acid. I told myself . . . "If I'm going to be puking all day, I'm at least going to have something besides vile stomach lining coming back out." Then I drank some water and ate a few saltines. I tried to get my shit together . . . mentally and physically.

Mind over matter was working, and I began to feel ok. I took the next shift. I had convinced my mind and my body that I was fine. And unbelievably, I was. At least, for now. But my potato was close by . . . just in case. I took the next four-hour shift from 14:00 to 18:00. The captain took over from 18:00 to midnight. And this time, I willed myself to sleep and rest.

Challenges Sailing with Dogs
Thursday, 13 September 2018 - THE ENGLISH CHANNEL
LEG 2 - DAY 3 AT SEA

At midnight, I was rested and ready for my night watch. The captain was exhausted. I could see it. He briefed me and went down to crash.

Meanwhile, we are still trying to get the dogs potty trained onboard. Sometimes they go to the bow and do their thing on the fake grass mat, but sometimes it's just too rough for them to be out there. And sometimes it's too rough for us to take them out there. I decided to move the grass mat into the cockpit and see if they might get the hint that it's ok to go in the cockpit. We just didn't want them going in the main cabin where we sleep.

So, I put the mat in the cockpit and Cap'n Jack immediately flooded the mat with pee. So, he was rewarded with the opportunity to go down below and cuddle in the warm cabin. But poor little Scout had not peed since we left the port, at least we had not seen her do it. And I just knew her little bladder was about to burst. I made her stay in the cockpit with me, and I think she went the whole six hours without going. There is a chance she went at some point, and I just didn't see her. I think that's what happened, but I'm not sure. Anyway, she joined me for the entire shift.

It was an extremely black night, but there were tons of stars sparkling in the sky lighting the way. Again, there was not a lot of traffic. I was able to relax enough to listen to an audible book.

By 06:00 I was ready for sleep. It was a long shift, but I wanted to let the captain sleep a little. I'm not sure if Scout ever pottied in the cockpit, but I let her crawl into bed with me anyway. She was so cuddly and sweet.

I woke up about four hours later and was feeling a bit icky, but I fought it. We were now on English waters and had raised the British ensign flag around sunrise. I asked if this meant we could now speak English. It's important to keep your sense of humor.

I was starving. I had been on a steady diet of gummy bears and saltines for the past couple days, and

I wanted us both to have a warm meal. We were still rocking a little and tilting, but I attempted to make some scrambled eggs. It's always a challenge to cook and balance, but I guess I'm getting better at it. I was motivated to put some real food in our bellies.

Falling in Love with The English Channel

As I returned to the cockpit, we realized that this was the farthest offshore we have been without seeing land and for the longest time. We could sort of see England to our starboard side, but only through the binoculars and only faintly. This was completely wide-open ocean. It's odd when you think about it. If you look on a map, The English Channel looks very narrow compared with other bodies of water. But it's 100 nautical miles at its widest point. When you are in the middle of it, all you can see is water and the horizon in your 360-degree view.

The English Channel is amazing. It is part of the Atlantic Ocean and separates the island of Britain from northern France, joining the North Sea to the Atlantic. It is approximately 350 miles long and is one of the busiest shipping lanes on the planet.

On this day, everything was grey—the sky, the water, everything. The only color we could see that wasn't a shade of grey was *Seefalke's* bright orange body sailing along at a steady 20-degree tilt. I had no idea the date on the calendar or even the day of the week. No idea. Day turned into night and night turned into day, and we just kept sailing along through the magnificent and sometimes eerie English Channel.

We still had no connection to the outside world except for family and friends who were communicating with us via text through our satellite GPS tracker. Our friends Dean and Tom were sending us weather and wind reports hourly, which was really cool and helpful! It was like they were right there with us!

Other than the colorless landscape, it was a beautiful day. The sun was shining directly into my face and sparkling off the water. I already had a little headache. Squinting at the sun was making it worse. Also, my toe was still throbbing. My head began to throb in sync with my toe and soon the head throbbing turned into a pounding.

What to do When You Don't Feel Well at Sea

I felt feverish and congested. I felt achy all over . . . like I was getting the flu. The captain thought perhaps I was having a little sun stroke, which is also possible. I was afraid to take Ibuprofen or Sudafed because I didn't want to upset my tummy. But I decided to take the chance and fight the oncoming illness with meds and continue to mentally fight any possible seasickness.

I decided to take another two-hour nap, but we were on such a heavy tilt that I felt like I was battling to hold on the entire time. It was not restful at all. I reluctantly returned to the cockpit for my 14:00 shift. Usually, I don't mind the tilt. It means that the winds are right and that we are making good speed. But at this point, I was having a really bad day, and I was just pissed at the tilt.

I was also wrestling a bit with my some of my feelings about being at sea for however many days and nights we had been out there at this point. I truly do love it most of the time, but I would be lying if I said I loved it all of the time. I started to feel guilty for feeling this way. I know I just wasn't feeling well. But mentally and physically, this particular voyage was just taking a toll on me.

My head was throbbing. I was frustrated with trying to stay balanced. By sore toe was pressing against the end of my boot causing pain that couldn't even compete with the headache and feverish aching. My ankles started to hurt, also from the balancing act. I was wrapped up in a full-on pity party and found myself wondering what the hell I was doing out there.

The captain never feels like this. He loves it all the time, at least that's what he says. He ignores the discomfort and the pain and just enjoys the challenge and the experience. I guess I'm just not there yet, and I have to be honest with myself that sometimes this is just not comfortable and fun. It is most of the time. But sometimes, it's just not.

I was also missing companionship. I know this sounds crazy since we are together 24/7. But when we are sailing in shifts, I'm sleeping when he's awake, and he's sleeping when I'm awake. We are like two ships that pass in the night.

I was reaching my statute of limitations on days at sea and fighting the 20-degree (sometimes 25-

degree) tilt was making me stiff and tense, worsening the already pounding headache.

I felt weak—both physically and mentally. I was letting physical discomfort creep into my brain and affect me mentally.

Finding the Inspiration to Keep Sailing

While I was focusing on all the pain and icky-ness, I started to think about Cheryl Strayed. I read her book "Wild" about four years ago and also saw the movie. She was dealing with the death of her mother, a divorce, and fighting drug addiction when she decided to punt her life and just start walking, all by herself. She hiked 1,100 miles alone along the Pacific Crest Trail on a quest to re-start her life and find peace and contentment. It was her book that inspired me to abandon the life I was living at the time in Birmingham, Alabama. I decided to sell the house I had lived in for 23 years and moved to Gulf Shores. I wanted to be near the water that gives me so much peace and happiness.

The things I remember the most about her book were her struggles—not her accomplishments. She fought the demons inside herself and came out cleaner and happier on the other side. She didn't love every day of her journey. But she didn't stop. She didn't give up. She kept going.

And, so will I.

By the end of my shift, I was really struggling.

SAILING THE ENGLISH CHANNEL LEG 2 - DAY 4 AT SEA
Friday, 14 September 2018

At midnight I woke up and decided to be strong. The captain told me to wake him in two hours. I told myself I could make it at least four.

The night was black. There were no stars. Just black . . . kind of like my mood. I wondered if other sailors ever felt this way—burned out just a little on the passion. Even too much of a good thing can sometimes be too much. Right?

I was still feverish. My face was hot, but the rest of my body had chills. I had a scratchy throat and was achy all over.

But soon the stars came out and filled the clearing sky. Some were as bright as the ships on the horizon. I relaxed and breathed in the fresh salt air as the cold wind cooled my hot face. I was completely soothed by the sound of the waves. I had taken my shift even though I didn't feel like it, and I was glad I did. Just like that, I felt free and happy again.

And I remembered why I do this.

After my two-hour shift that I stretched to four hours, the captain took over at 04:00 and I finally got a few hours of sound sleep. I had stopped moping and whining about the bad stuff and began to embrace the good things.

We began to reach the end of the English Channel where the opening of The North Atlantic begins. All of a sudden, the grey water turned a deep navy blue. It was amazing as brilliant shades of color began to burst onto the horizon—like in the Wizard of Oz movie when everything transforms from black-and-white to color. There were birds flying everywhere, and we could see the gorgeous French coastline to our left.

The heavy waves were no longer choppy and uncomfortable. They were still about three-meters high, but they were longer and smoother and softer. They looked like a warm blanket rolling toward us. We were cruising along relatively even at this point . . . without much tilt. The waves were no longer lifting us out of the air and slamming us back down onto the water. They were now raising us ever-so-calmly and then gently setting us down as if we were made of glass.

All four of us sat on the deck and rode the waves for a long time.

Sailing and Sea Life

A school of dolphins greeted us just as we crossed the line where The English Channel ends and the open Northern Atlantic begins. They intentionally swam right toward us and then played in the wake of *Seefalke's* bow for about five minutes.

As often as I see dolphins at home in Bon Secour Bay, I never get tired of seeing them. They are like old friends, but each time is like the first time. I am always excited to see them. This was kind of like that, but a bit different. I didn't know these dolphins and they were huge—at least twice the size of our hometown dolphins—and so playful.

The water was deep—more than 90 meters—but you could see clearly as the dolphins swam and played underneath *Seefalke* and all around us.

Then they just swam away. As quickly as they had appeared, they disappeared into the deep blue sea. It's moments like this that stay with you forever.

And again, I remembered why I do this.

TIPS FROM CHAPTER 5

- Spread your legs shoulder-width apart, bend your knees, and perform a slow-motion, hula-hoop action with the lower part of your body to cushion and balance the movement.
- Carefully plan your passage. Try to determine just the right time for departure to best take advantage of the weather, wind, currents, and conditions. Then determine the best route, remembering that the conditions could change at any time at sea.
- Remember that it's the hard parts of sailing that make it special. If it were easy, anyone could do it.
- Delay the departure if you are feeling rushed, or stressed, or if you have other injuries that are bothering you.
- Sometimes mind over matter is the best cure. Try not to think about the queasiness, if possible.
- Try to focus on the beauty surrounding you— the sunset, the colors, the scenery, etc. This will help to take your mind off of the uneasiness.

- Remember that seasickness is not your fault. Don't get mad at yourself or frustrated when it sets in. Instead, focus on ways to quell the effects. Frustration will only make it worse.
- Try to find something to distract you, like listening to an audible book or music.
- Try to keep your sense of humor and find ways to relax and laugh with other crew members.
- At times when you are feeling ok, try to cook something to have a warm, substantial meal in your belly, if at all possible.
- Try not to squint at the sun. This could cause a headache, which could lead to seasickness.
- Sometimes taking an antihistamine will help to clear the sinuses and help you to avoid seasickness.
- Try to avoid having a pity party and focusing on all the ways you feel bad. Try to find something positive to think about. Physical discomfort can creep into your psyche and make you convince yourself you feel worse.
- Whether it's the challenge or the joy of sailing, the scenery or the wildlife, remember why you do this so you will know that the bouts with seasickness are worth it!

CHAPTER 6

When There Are No Calm Waters – Sailing the Bay of Biscay

My experiences with seasickness in The Baltic were rough, but these were one-day sails. This meant that we could sail forward knowing that at the end of the day, we had a marina or an anchorage waiting for us. Rest and recovery were always just a few hours away.

Multiple-day passages are much tougher. The seasickness can last into the night watches and throw the schedule into a whirl as chaotic as the motion causing the uneasiness.

As we began planning our worldwide voyage, my greatest fear was never crossing the Atlantic. For me, it was crossing the Bay of Biscay. I made the mistake of researching this remarkable body of water—a bit too much research, perhaps.

Sometimes, too much knowledge can lead to more fear. From my online logbook, read these entries that first describe my anticipation of the dreaded Biscay, and then chronicle the day-by-day experience of my worst-ever bout with seasickness and how I survived it.

What is the Bay of Biscay?

Ernest Hemingway once said:

"There is no joy in the journey's end if there is no joy in the journey."

Life is supposed to be about the journey, not the destination. Right?

As I prepared for a sailing passage across the infamous Bay of Biscay, I began to question that theory for the first time in five decades.

I decided to focus on the destination—Spain. I had never been there, and I always wanted to go. Now I had the opportunity! It's the power of positive thinking. Right? I continued to brush up on my Spanish and think about the pintxos and the paella, the historic sights, and the sunny beaches.

It was important to stop thinking about what it would take to get there in a tiny little sailboat.

Ok, I couldn't help but think about it a little.

Frankly, I was terrified.

Why Does the Bay of Biscay Have Such a Bad Reputation?

Seriously, crossing the Bay of Biscay was the only part of our worldwide sailing voyage that had me shaking in my skin. It's been called "The Valley of Death," "The Vomiting Venus," and "The Trunk of the Atlantic U-Boat Menace." Jane Russell, author of "The Atlantic Crossing Guide," was seasick for eight days while crossing the Bay of Biscay. This was the first thing I read when I began studying her book about a year before my cross-Atlantic sailing voyage. I worried about the Bay of Biscay every day for a solid year.

The Bay of Biscay is a gulf located in the Celtic Sea of the northwest Atlantic Ocean between the northern coast of Spain and the western coast of France. The average depth is 1,745 meters and the maximum depth is 4,890 meters. There are also many dangerous shallow areas.

Some of the fiercest weather conditions of the Atlantic Ocean happen in the Bay of Biscay. It is home to large storms during the winter months, and there have been countless shipwrecks that have resulted from the gruesome weather. Depressions enter the Bay from the West. They dry out and then are born again as thunderstorms that look like hurricanes and crash into the Bay. When the wind and waves come in from different directions, they can collide and create confused water inside the Bay.

Many sailors describe this as like being inside a washing machine.

Huge Atlantic swells can form near the coast, making many ports inaccessible. Because of the extreme weather in the winter, there are abnormally high waves at times.

The Bay of Biscay has been feared by seamen dating back to the beginning of the second World War when German U-boats ruled the area, and many American and British ships sank in her waters.

Getting Mentally Ready for a
Bay of Biscay Sailing Passage

We sat in Brittany, France at Camaret sur Mer for nine days awaiting just the right weather window. This gave me perhaps too much time to think about and fear the Bay of Biscay. The first few days we were there, we enjoyed warm, sunny weather, and we had a great time exploring the area.

But the days leading to our departure, we sat inside our bright orange, steel-constructed vessel, *Seefalke*, waiting out harsh weather that had been passing through. This didn't help with my mental preparation.

It was stormy and rainy and very windy for several days, but we hunkered down inside *Seefalke's* belly—warm and cozy and safe. It felt like what I imagine it would feel like to live inside a submarine. We could hear water echoing as the waves lapped against *Seefalke's* steel hull. We didn't go outside much during those pre-departure storms, opting instead for the dry shelter of our bright orange cocoon. We were securely tied to the pier but rocked and swayed as if we were at sea. We could hear the angry wind howling outside.

This was the good news...

- We had a favorable weather window, a solid passage plan that took nine days to develop, and a patient crew that would never take any unnecessary chances.
- Our 43-foot ketch was built for this kind of blue water sailing. It has a four-foot deep cockpit in the

center of the boat, which protects us completely from all sides. It has two masts with adjustable sails in many sizes to cushion the blows of heavy gusts and gale-force winds.

- There was an opportunity to see some cool sea wildlife. Many different species of whales and dolphins can be seen in the Bay of Biscay, including beaked whales, minke whales, fin whales, harbor porpoises, short-beaked common dolphins, striped dolphins, long-finned pilot whales, sperm whales, and the northern bottlenose whale. Scaleless dragonfish are native to the Bay of Biscay.
- We had a passage plan that basically puts us on a straight course directly to A Caruña, Spain.
- I was ready to explore Spain for the first time!

Ok, so maybe I shouldn't totally discount the journey. Perhaps I should embrace the opportunity and the challenge to be among those brave enough to sail on this incredible and challenging body of water. With exciting Spanish lands to explore on the other side, I had the opportunity to face another fear and challenge myself in ways I never thought possible. Perhaps there is joy in the journey, after all!

"Twenty years from now you will be more disappointed by the things that you didn't do than by the ones you did do. So, throw off the bowlines. Sail away from the safe harbor. Catch the trade winds in your sails. Explore. Dream. Discover." – Mark Twain

Battling Seasickness Through the Bay of Biscay

The Bay of Biscay is located somewhere at the corner of your wildest dream-come-true and your worst possible nightmare.

You dread it, and you look forward to it—all at the same time. As it approaches, anticipation sets in. Then your excitement competes heavily with your fear—a fear you can't quite convince yourself is not really there no matter how hard you try. The battle of conflicting emotions is like a rivalry football game that goes into five overtimes. The competition is neck and neck until the end, and you are never quite sure who will win the battle. It's anyone's ballgame.

My experience crossing the infamous Bay of Biscay tapped into every possible emotion—even a few that I didn't realize I had. I battled extreme fatigue, gut-wrenching seasickness, dehydration, and muscles so sore I barely had the strength to even hang on while *Seefalke* was surfing violently on the sometimes 12-foot waves. But in the end, we made it through to sunny, beautiful A Caruña, Spain. I'm not sure I can remember a time in my life that I felt so physically and mentally challenged . . . and accomplished.

It's kind of like having a baby. Women experience brutal pain and discomfort during pregnancy and especially during childbirth. We put our bodies through extreme torture to create this tiny human that immediately gives us so much joy. With time, we can't even remember what it took to get from the gruesome nightmare to the most remarkable dream-come-true. I believe this is how it's possible for women to have more than one child. With time, you forget the pain and only remember the fantastic reward that completely overshadows the difficult journey required to get there.

This experience doesn't even come close to the joy of motherhood. But I can tell you that it was something like that—the personal reward of making it to the end of the Bay of Biscay greatly outweighs the struggle.

DAY 1 Challenging Bay of Biscay Sailing Passage

Monday, 24 September 2018 - DEPARTURE FROM CAMARET SUR MER - 11:15

Our original plan was to get through the Bay of Biscay by the end of August. With all our delays getting *Seefalke* ready for her blue-water voyage, we missed that mark by a long shot.

It is not recommended for small leisure craft like *Seefalke* to cross the bay in the winter months. It's not really a fun time for huge heavy freighters, either. There are ships much larger and heavier than *Seefalke* sitting at the bottom of the Bay of Biscay's 4,860-meter-deep waters. Don't think for a second this wasn't on my mind.

We were lucky. We waited patiently for nine days in the Camaret sur Mer port in Brittany, France and finally found an opening—a pocket in which we would have northeasterly winds for four straight days. This would push us on a direct course with minimal wind changes all the way down to A Caruña, Spain.

It was our best chance, and we took it.

It was magnificently beautiful as we departed and began sailing into the Celtic Sea. The sun was shining brightly. The scenery was spectacular! We could clearly see the French coastline. Waves crashed against the gorgeous rock formations along the cliffs that gave us a strong wind shadow and protected us for a short time from the open sea—a very short time.

I asked the skipper when we would officially be inside the Bay of Biscay. His response: "You'll know it when we are there."

A school of common dolphins swam toward *Seefalke* and played with us for a long time. The waters were so calm I actually lie on the deck with the pups and took a short nap as the hot sun kissed my skin. I was completely relaxed.

But something deep inside warned me not to expect this for long.

About an hour before sunset, the waves began to swell, and the wind grew stronger. At this point, the waves were rolling in from the Atlantic at only about 2 meters (6 feet) high. But I knew it—it was obvious we were now in the Bay of Biscay. The waves were already rocking the 11-ton *Seefalke* forcefully from side to side.

There was no land in sight—only the deep blue sea.

How to Mentally Survive the Bay of Biscay

It's at this point that you realize there is no going back. You are in the middle of the open ocean. There is nowhere to stop for at least three or four more days. It's too deep to drop an anchor. You are committed. There is no choice but to push forward all the way to Spain.

There is some traffic in the Bay of Biscay, but we fortunately didn't see much. The wind was strong but steady and coming from the perfect direction. The waves were getting larger—already some were 3 meters (9 feet), but they were pushing us mostly from behind. These were as perfect conditions as we could possibly hope for in the Bay of Biscay in winter. We decided we would sail in regular 4-hour shifts.

The captain took the first watch from 20:00 to midnight. I went down into the cabin with our four-legged crew—Cap'n Jack and Scout—and tried to sleep. We were on a heavy heel to the starboard side. The dogs were secure in their barricaded bunk and didn't seem to want to even try to join me in mine. My regular bunk is on the port side, so there was a feeling of constant sliding down to the right. It was like trying to sleep on a very slippery, slanted block of ice. I tried to get up at one point to re-position myself when a huge wave rocked *Seefalke* and threw me to the other side of the cabin. Hard. I banged the back of my head on a cabinet while my shoulder blades crashed against the corner of the cabinet.

I tried to find a comfortable position to rest, but it wasn't easy. I had to bury my arm underneath the mattress to support myself from sliding and also had to leverage my right leg against the bunk on the opposite side of the cabin.

Nothing was flying across the cabin. Everything on the outside was secure, finally. But as I tried to relax, I could hear so many things moving around inside the cabinets. I could hear pots and pans banging against each other. I could hear forks and spoons being shuffled around inside one cabinet. All the coffee cups and dishes were being tossed around. *Seefalke* was being shaken like a martini. It was loud and annoying, and felt like I was inside a haunted house full of drunken, rowdy ghosts rattling heavy chains determined to prevent me from sleeping.

I got no rest.

How to Battle Seasickness in the Bay of Biscay
DAY 2 Bay of Biscay Passage
Tuesday, 25 September 2018

I took my shift at midnight. Again, this is one of those times when the sweet dream intersects into a nightmare. On the one hand, it was a gorgeous night—clear, black skies with millions of bright, sparkling stars. There was a full moon casting a brilliant spotlight onto the gigantic waves. Sometimes, I would look behind me at a huge wave rolling in and see a couple dolphins surfing in the wave.

It was so cool!

On the other hand . . . it was terrifying!

When you see a huge, swelling wave coming toward you, your first reaction is, "Wow! This is so beautiful!" Before you can even get the words out of your mouth, that same wave slams against the side of your ship's bright orange hull. The freezing cold saltwater drenches you and throws you violently to the other side of the cockpit with so much force you can barely catch yourself.

At least with the bright moon lighting our way, I could see the waves rolling in which gave me a chance to brace myself before contact. We always wear life vests, but we also strap ourselves in the cockpit in these kinds of conditions. And with *Seefalke's* four-foot deep, center cockpit, we are protected on all sides. There is a feeling of safety and security. For this I'm grateful. But for 240 straight minutes, I stood in the middle of the cockpit with my legs spread a little more than shoulder width to balance myself, and I just held on with both hands as tightly as I could. It's pretty much all I could do.

Meanwhile, the captain and the pups slept comfortably below.

It's so interesting how some sailors can turn off their ears. They can hear the slightest flap in the sail from a deep sound sleep, but the clankety-clanking pots and pans and silverware tossing around in the cabinets don't bother them at all.

When I went back down at 04:00 I was exhausted. I couldn't do anything about the heavy waves and the rocking sailboat, but I decided to do something about the clankety-clanking in the cabinets. I grabbed six huge fluffy beach towels and began stuffing them into the cabinets to try to cushion the tossing around of all the stuff. For the most part this solved the problem, although I spent the next three days continuing to make adjustments to this system.

Meanwhile, I simply could not sleep comfortably on the bunk with the heavy tilt and rocking boat. And I needed some sleep. Desperately.

I thought about crawling into the other bunk with the pups, but this would cause discomfort issues of a different kind. Their area is small, and I would have to curl up into the fetal position and also share the space with them and all the dog hair. I thought about moving into the stern cabin, but I didn't want to leave Cap'n Jack and Scout. They were doing fine, but I could tell they were a little afraid. I just didn't want to leave them.

So, I got creative.

There is a narrow walkway between the two bunks. I threw down a sleeping bag and crawled onto the floor. This was perfect. I had both bunks to cushion the motion and protect me from sliding in either direction. It was like I was in a baby cradle. It was still rocking, but at least I wasn't being slung all over the cabin. I could sleep without having to hold on to something, and for me this was perfect. At some point during that shift, the pups joined me. I awoke with four velvety Beagle ears tickling my face. I finally got a little sleep and returned to the cockpit at 08:00 for my next shift.

The waves were HUGE at this point—some of them were 4-meters (12-feet) high. And they were constant. Sometimes when you are sailing you have a period of heavy waves and then there are breaks with calm smooth waters. But we had zero breaks from the waves. They just kept coming. Sometimes they were 2 meters, sometimes 3 meters and sometimes 4 meters.

But they were ALWAYS there. The wind was blowing at a steady 20 to 28 knots the entire time with occasional gusts of more than 30 knots. It was like this for three straight days.

About 30 minutes into this shift, I was still settling in and trying to find a comfortable balancing position. I saw a few dolphins flipping around in *Seefalke's* wake. This was just so cool! I never get tired of seeing them! Scout came up to the cockpit for a quick potty, and it was nice to have her with me. The pups are such good company, especially when we are working in shifts and are never awake at the same time for several days. It can get lonely. Cap'n Jack and Scout are not very good conversationalists, but they are great listeners! I find myself just talking and talking and talking to them. They don't seem to mind.

At around 09:30, I could feel my belly begin to contract. All of a sudden, I felt weak and dizzy—and nauseous. *Oh, no. Please don't let me be seasick!*

I reached for my potato with my left hand and began reciting the Greek Alphabet to distract me (those of you who regularly read this blog know that this can help with my seasickness).

But it was too late.

I leaned over the port side sea rail while everything inside my belly spewed out of my mouth with great force. It still amazes me how the seasickness can be so forceful. My entire body contracts and jerks me from my feet. With each heave I can feel my limbs become lifeless. It rips away all your strength. It holds your will to live hostage at gunpoint. You just can't move.

Meanwhile, while leaning over the sea rail completely helpless, the massive 3-to-4-meter waves continue to roll in. The wind still blows forcefully at around 25 knots. I was holding on to the winch drum for support between heaves. Generally, when the seasickness hits me, it's just the end of any possibility of being productive after that—at least until the waters begin to calm. But this time, I knew there was no way that one sailor could easily handle the Bay of Biscay alone in these heavy conditions for two more days and two more nights. I just had to keep going.

At noon, the captain awakened and was going to come up for his shift. He was feeling as badly as me, and I wanted to stay in the fresh air. So, I told him if he wanted to sleep some more, it was ok. I wasn't going anywhere. I couldn't leave my little corner of the cockpit, or my grip on the winch drum.

He slept another hour then joined me. I wanted to stay in the fresh, cool air because that was helping a little. I tried to lie on the cockpit bench, but it was too hard to hang on. After two more hours, I finally gave in and went down to sleep in the cradle on the floor.

Each shift got more and more difficult.

At this point, the waves and the wind were at their heaviest. I was green and weak and feverish. My face was broiling hot. A whole sack of potatoes couldn't help me now. And even if they could, I couldn't let go of my grip. I didn't have a spare hand with which to hold one. My arms and shoulders were aching from constantly holding on and trying to maintain balance.

The captain was suffering too, and the dogs seemed uncomfortable. We decided we would take two-hour shifts through the night because four hours was just too much for either of us in these conditions. This meant shorter spurts of sleep, but a bit less brutal for the helmsman.

For me, through the entire night each shift was like déjà vu all over again.

Sail, puke, sleep, repeat.

Sail, puke, sleep, repeat.

But the bright full moon continued to light our way.

Battling Dehydration and Seasickness
DAY 3 Bay of Biscay Passage
Wednesday, 26 September 2018

My stomach was empty. In the past 24 hours I had eaten nothing but half a gummy bear, which I threw up before I could try to make an effort to eat the other half.

On my next morning shift, I awoke to knotty charley horses in my calves, back spasms, and a pounding headache. I felt so weak, my legs could barely support my own body weight. I knew the dehydration had set in. I needed to eat something and drink something.

I was able to slowly nibble away half a banana, half a cracker, and a few sips of water. This helped. It gave me just enough strength to throw it back up shortly after consuming it. I was feeling dreadful, but I knew I needed to push on.

I told myself that no matter how badly I felt, I would not miss a shift! This became my goal and my quest. And at this point, we only had one day and one night to go. We were on the home stretch.

Even while I was feeling so icky, I couldn't help but notice that it was such a beautiful day. Bright, clear, blue skies and an ocean as deep and vibrant blue as anything I could ever imagine. It was glorious!

We continued with four-hour shifts during the day and at around 17:30, something amazing happened!

I heard a loud blowing sound that sounded like a distant foghorn at first. I looked to the port side and through the gigantic waves I saw a huge grey form on the surface of the water that was at least three times the size of *Seefalke* and only about 30 meters away. I only saw it for a couple seconds and then saw only a huge grey tail splash in the air. I believe it was a sperm whale, but I'm not positive. It was definitely a whale. It was so close to us. And something told me we were going to make it.

I didn't have time to grab a camera, so I have no proof. You'll just have to believe me.

At this point, I was just grateful to be out there. I didn't care that I was sick and tired and hungry and hurting. I was lucky enough to see something that most people only see in other people's photos or movies. I searched the water to try and get another glimpse of this remarkable creature. But he was gone. As instantly as he had appeared, he had vanished into the deep blue sea.

I ate a whole banana and an apple and three crackers. I drank a little water. I wanted to get my strength back. I wanted to find a way to embrace this challenge and get to the end.

As expected, the food didn't stay with me long. It left me at around the same time the captain came up for his shift. But at least my insides didn't taste like stomach acid anymore.

Finding a Way to Make it Through the Bay of Biscay

DAY 4 Bay of Biscay Passage
Thursday, 27 September 2018

After another night of familiar four-hour shifts—sail, puke, sleep, repeat—I was awakened around 08:30 by an exhilarated skipper. "Get up here! I SEE LAND!"

I came charging up to the cockpit and almost burst into tears! It was way, way, way off in the distance. But yes, we could see Spain! We raised the Spanish courtesy flag, and it was glorious to see it flying high on our mast!

We were still about 7 hours away, but the end was in sight!

We began to see beautiful birds gracefully flying overhead and grazing along the surface of the water. I thought about the old sailors who were at sea for months and even years at a time. They didn't have weather-predicting technology, or GPS or other instrumentation to guide them—only a compass. Some of them would travel with a cage of ravens. They would release one and if it circled overhead, they knew that they were not close to land. But if the raven began to fly in a certain direction, they knew that land was near. The sailors would follow the flying bird toward land.

More dolphins greeted us and played in *Seefalke's* wake. Within a couple hours, after three straight days with no break from the nonstop heavy waves, the waters finally began to calm a bit. All of a sudden, we were floating on a sea of glass. It was so clear and smooth I could see my reflection in the water.

We were trying not to celebrate too much. Sailors are very superstitious, after all. I thought about the challenge and about the adventure. As bad as it was, it was the best possible conditions we could have ever asked for during this time of year. The wind was always coming from the right direction. We didn't have to tack or change directions. We had a straight course all the way to our destination. The waves were behind us or beside us and never against us. The sun was always shining. We had a full moon to light our way every night. There were no storms or squalls.

I was beginning to see the positive side of things.

The captain told me he was proud of me. He doesn't hand out compliments very often. It's just not his style. This made me proud. I was proud of myself. As bad as I felt almost the entire time, I never missed a shift.

With the calm waters, my appetite began to return. We still had about four hours to go, so I went down and cooked some pasta so we could put some warm, solid food in our bellies.

But our challenges weren't over yet.

A very heavy fog began to roll in. We saw a huge freighter in front of us and the top half of this gigantic ship was hidden completely by the fog. Soon, the ship disappeared from the surface of the sea completely. It just wasn't there anymore. It was eerie. Once again, the wonderful dream was interrupted briefly for a bit of a nightmare.

Soon the fog was all around us. We literally could not see five feet in front of us. Zero visibility. And worse, other ships could not see us.

We received AIS signals on the plotter that there were three ships close to us. We could hear their loud, long foghorns blowing in the distance. We could tell one was in front of us, and two off to the starboard side. But we couldn't see them at all. And we had no idea how far away from us they were. They blasted long horn signals. We blasted long horn signals.

If there is restricted visibility, ships are required to blast their horn every two minutes. If you are using the motor, the signal required is a long, eight-second blast. If you are under sail, the signal is one long blast followed by two short blasts. We kept blasting away and just held our breath hoping that we would all avoid each other.

Soon the fog lifted, and we could see again. The Spanish coastline was coming into focus and bursting with vibrant color.

It feels incredible to finally be in Spain. In the next weeks, we will sail to several ports in Spain and Portugal on our way to Morocco!

This is the thing about nightmares. You eventually wake up. The nightmare is now over and the dream of making it through the Bay of Biscay is a reality. From the beginning, I feared this passage. At times I couldn't even think about it without having a bit of a panic attack. I warned my family and friends to avoid Googling the Bay of Biscay until after we had crossed it.

We met one sailor in Helgoland who told us he sailed The Bay of Biscay with his wife during the winter, and she has threatened to divorce him ever since.

Now it's in our backwater.

I'm glad we did it, and I feel an incredible sense of accomplishment. But I'm not sure I ever want to birth a Bay of Biscay baby ever again! At least that's how I feel today. Ask me again tomorrow, and the answer may be different.

TIPS FROM CHAPTER 6

- Arm yourself with information but try to avoid doing too much research about bodies of water or conditions that scare you.
- Try to enjoy the journey by focusing on the good parts and think about the excitement of the destination rather than the difficulty of the passage.
- Mentally prepare for challenging passages so you can be prepared and quell the fear.
- Don't take any unnecessary chances with the weather or conditions. Wait patiently for the perfect weather window before departing.

- When you see huge waves headed your way, try to brace yourself before contact to prevent excessive movement.
- When captain and crew are seasick, shorten the shifts (for example, from four hours to two hours).
- Find a comfortable place in the cabin to sleep— one in which you won't be tossed around too much (for example, on the floor between the bunks).
- Don't try to cook in rough conditions. Instead, prepare in advance some snacks and cold meals and have them available to grab and eat quickly in the cockpit.
- Have plenty of drinks available in the cockpit to stay hydrated.
- Prepare a thermos of ginger tea before departing and keep it handy in the cockpit in case the queasiness sets in.
- When you feel the uneasiness set in, try to distract yourself with something that requires concentration (for example, recite the Greek Alphabet, count to 100 in German, sing or recite all the lyrics of a song, recite dialogue from your favorite movie). In other words, distract your brain.
- Challenge yourself. (For example, I made it a goal to never miss a shift, no matter how bad I felt). This will give you something to strive for and a happy feeling of accomplishment.
- Find something to hold on to for balance (for example, a winch drum).

CHAPTER 7

Is It All in Your Head? The Psychology of Seasickness

I'll say it again, I'm not a doctor. I'm also not a psychologist. But I'm convinced that seasickness is at least somewhat psychological.

Many experts agree.

In his book, Psychological Mechanisms That Exacerbate Motion Sickness (Dobie, 2019), Thomas Dobie's research shows that "individuals whose careers are in jeopardy are most likely to have an arousal overlay when confronted with a provocative motion environment. Motion sickness is also likely to affect people if they have had a previous uncomfortable motion experience."

He says that this doesn't mean that motion sickness is entirely psychological, but instead he suggests that there is a psychological component. For example, a motion sickness episode can often happen based on the memory of previous motion discomfort. He also believes the situation is made worse by high achievers.

I believe there is some "muscle memory" involved based on a personal experience. Several months after my year-long sailing adventure, I took a short cruise on a 24-foot motorboat with my daughter,

Shelby, and an experienced and licensed boat captain, Donnie Vinson of Team Vinson Charters.

I had been on this boat with Captain Donnie several times and had not had any bouts with seasickness onboard. He's an experienced and conscientious boat captain, and we had never had severe weather or gone too far offshore. On this day, we cruised to about 30 miles offshore in the Gulf of Mexico, fishing for red snapper.

We reached his honey hole, and he steadied the boat. It was a warm sunny, summer day, but there were about 1-to-2-foot choppy waves. After experiencing 12-to-16-foot waves in the Bay of Biscay, I couldn't imagine that these little waves would affect me at all.

About halfway to the fishing spot, I began to think about some of my epic bouts with seasickness. The thoughts were creeping into my head as we began to lose sight of land, but I told myself, *"Hey, there is nothing to worry about. I've crossed the Atlantic Ocean in a tiny sailboat. I've crossed the Bay of Biscay in a tiny sailboat. I was hundreds and even thousands of miles offshore in super high waves. This is nothing compared with that. Right?"*

Shelby and Captain Donnie dropped their lines and immediately began pulling in gorgeous, huge Alabama Red Snapper. I felt a bit rocky and a little queasy and did what I shouldn't do. I sat down and surrendered to the feeling. Rather than focusing on the horizon or distracting my brain, I let myself feel green and icky. Shelby and Captain Donnie felt fine.

I lie on the boat's floor for the rest of the day, including the ride back to shore. I threw up a few times and felt horrible and awful the entire day. I'm convinced that the conditions were nowhere near as rough and rocky as those I had experienced previously. But I'm also convinced that it was some sort of muscle memory of previous bouts with seasickness that had entered my psyche and caused the episode.

I reminded myself that sailors much more experienced than me suffer from seasickness. Still, it frustrates me that I'm a victim of this phenomenon, even when the conditions are mild.

It helps to know that I'm not alone.

"The misery I endured from sea-sickness is far far beyond what I ever guessed at," Charles Darwin once wrote to his father. "If it was not for sea-sickness, the whole world would be sailors."

Even farther back, Greek physician Hippocrates presaged our current term, "motion sickness," writing, "sailing on the sea proves that motion disorders the body." (Beck, 2015)

So, is it all in our heads?

One study found that motion sickness can be reduced through visuospatial training, which involves a person manipulating 3D objects in their imagination. (Huzar, 2020)

Another study proved that "Motion sickness is a well-known nausea and vomiting syndrome in otherwise healthy people. The physical signs of motion sickness occur in both humans and animals during travel by sea, automobile or airplane and in space. Furthermore, some other special situations, such as simulators, the cinema and video games, have been described as causing pseudomotion sickness."

The study further found that "Motion sickness is considered a physiological vertigo and is not a true sickness in the strict sense of the word but rather is a normal response to an abnormal situation.

"Motion sickness is caused by certain types of motion and is induced during passive locomotion in vehicles, generated by unfamiliar body accelerations, to which the person has not adapted, or by an intersensory conflict between vestibular and visual stimuli. Motion sickness indiscriminately affects air, sea, road and space travelers. All individuals (humans and animals) possessing an intact vestibular apparatus can get motion sickness given the right quality and quantity of provocative stimulation, although there are wide and consistent individual differences in the degree of susceptibility." (Schmal, 2013)

So, I ask the questions, can we really "train our brains" to be less susceptible to motion sickness? Is it really just psychological?

I'm convinced there is a psychological component, but if you've ever experienced the effects of seasickness like Darwin and me, you have to believe it's very, very physical as well!

TIPS FROM CHAPTER 7

- Stress can be a psychological trigger for motion sickness. When in a provocative motion situation, try to relax and not think about stressors like your job.
- Try not to think about past bouts with seasickness when you are on a boat or in a

situation that causes extreme motion. Try to fight the feeling rather than surrendering to it so quickly.

- Some studies show that visuospatial training can help quell the effects of motion sickness.

CHAPTER 8

Battling Seasickness with Pharmaceuticals

Pharmaceuticals do work for many people who struggle with seasickness, but I am an exception. Trust me, I tried every medication out there. Meds simply did not work for me. Most important, on a two-person crew, it's impossible to take a pill that may make you sleep for many hours. We were generally on four-hour shifts and often on two-hour shifts, so medications that make you drowsy were simply not an option for me.

However, yes, medications do work for many sailors and others who struggle with motion sickness or seasickness. I can't provide a comprehensive book about battling seasickness without a chapter about these options.

Please remember that I am not a doctor, and I am not prescribing or recommending ANY of these medications.

Based on my research and on some meds that I've tried, here is some information about pharmaceuticals that may help with seasickness or motion sickness. I do not recommend any of them. **Please consult a medical professional before trying any of these options.**

Please also remember that seasickness is often easier to avoid than to cure. Most remedies need to be taken a couple of hours before departure. Different treatments work better for different people, and they will affect different people in different ways. You may need to try a few to determine which is best for you.

Remember to check with your doctor to make sure that any remedy does not conflict with medication you are currently taking—prescription or over-the-counter.

Common Medications Used for Seasickness and Motion Sickness

Scopolamine patches, worn behind the ear like a tiny band-aid, are the most common prescription drugs for seasickness. Scopolamine also comes in pill form. The patches last up to three days, provide time-release doses of the drug, and are usually very effective for preventing nausea. (Garrison, 2019)

I personally tried these patches on a long passage from Morocco to the Canary Islands. For me, they only caused a severe headache, which ended up being worse that the seasickness. Also, they are expensive and required a prescription.

My general practitioner subscribed them for me, and they cost $50 for each patch. In the end, the cure can't be worse than the illness, so this remedy was not for me. However, I do know several sailors who use the patches and find that they are helpful.

Keep in mind that most medications for motion sickness need to be taken at least 30 minutes before exposure to the activity that can cause the problem. Some recommend taking two hours before departure. Everything I've read says that people with glaucoma or prostate problems should not take most of these medications unless advised by their doctor.

Research shows that individuals could avoid motion sickness by pretreating with klonopin and ondansetron. That being said, here are more details about motion sickness medications from health care professionals.

- *Meclizine (Antivert, Bonine)*. This is in the antihistamine family and can cause drowsiness. Like most other medications, it is best to take these before motion stimulation. Meclizine does not work for all types of motion—for example, coriolis stimulation. (Dornhoffer, 2004)
- *Dimenhydrinate* (Dramamine). This is similar to meclizine. Liquid forms are available for children 2 years of age or more.
- *Cyclizine* is similar to meclizine. It is suitable for children 6 years of age or older as well as adults. It is most useful in situations involving short trips (e.g. automobile).
- *Haldol, Thorazine*. These anti-psychotic drugs have dopamine blocking activity which is useful for blocking nausea as well as stimulating stomach motion which helps clear food from the digestive tract. These drugs probably work on the central motion sickness machinery rather than the vestibular system. (Hain, 2020)
- *Calcium channel blockers*. Reported cinnarizine—a mixed antihistamine/calcium channel blocker, to be very effective in preventing seasickness, when used in a 50 mg dose. (Shupak, 1994) This medication is not available in the United States. Flunarizine is a similar medication to cinnarizine (Lee JA, 1986) but it has more

dopamine blocking effect. As calcium channels appear to be important in the vestibular periphery, and these drugs are very sloppy, their action may simply be vestibular suppression. In the US, a combination of verapamil and meclizine would be likely to create a similar effect.

- *Promethazine*. This drug is one of the most effective available for motion sickness. (Dornhoffer, 2004) One dose lasts up to 8 hours. Like the other drugs, it can cause drowsiness. It is not appropriate for cognitive workers.

- *Diazepam (valium)* and related "benzodiazepine" medications such as lorazepam and klonazepam. While these drugs are not traditionally used for motion sickness, some people find them very useful in small amounts, typically taken about 30 minutes prior to motion exposure. Researchers say they have rarely encountered people who could not prevent motion sickness by taking a klonazepam 30 minutes prior to the exposure. On the other hand, one of these, lorazepam, did not help prevent motion sickness from coriolois stimulation (Dornhoffer, 2004). These medications are sedating and addictive. They probably work by suppressing central vestibular responses. Unless one is addicted and has developed tolerance, only small amounts of benzodiazepine medications are compatible with normal cognitive function.

- *Scopolamine patches* are sometimes very helpful. They are a time release form of an anticholinergic medication, scopolamine. Scopolamine is also available in pill format (usually given for irritable bowel). Scopolamine was found the most useful medication for prevention of motion sickness induced by cross-coriolis stimulation (Dornhoffer, 2004). Whether or not this is true for other types of motion stimulation is not known. Scopolamine contains both the D and L isomers of hyoscine. Scopolamine (hyoscine) is close, but not exactly the same as L-hyocyanime (the active ingredient in Levsin). Scopolamine may have more central activity while Levsin (a GI medication) less. In other words, Levsin is not equivalent to scopolamine. It is a close relative, however. Scopace is an oral version. Anticholinergics that do not penetrate the blood-brain barrier, such as robinul, would seem to be poor choices, as they have no target.
- *Ondansetron* and other serotonin-family anti-nausea drugs. These are powerful anti-nausea medications. They do not prevent motion sickness, but they may prevent vomiting. They work very well, with almost no side effects at all. In general, they are an excellent choice for nausea.
- *Migraine medications*: Verapamil (a calcium channel blocker), venlafaxine (an antidepressant, in this context used as a migraine prevention medication). Doctors favor verapamil as it is also

useful in cyclic vomiting. Triptans have been reported as mildly helpful in preventing motion sickness in persons with migraine. (Furman, 2011) There are not any known reports concerning the longer acting triptans such as frovatriptan or naratriptan, which would seem to be logical picks.

- *Seizure medications phenytoin and carbamazepine* (sodium channel blockers). Phenytoin (Knox GW, 1994) would seem to be a very bad choice due to its difficulty in dosing. Carbamazepine also would seem to us to be a bad choice due to significant risk of side effects. Doctors are not sure about safer agents such as oxcarbamazine and are dubious about this group but have occasionally had good results.

Medications that do not work for motion sickness:

Antihistamines such as fexofenadine and cetirizine that do not get into the brain (Bob Cheung, 2001) are not effective for motion sickness. It also seems very unlikely that anticholinergics that don't get into the brain (such as Robinul) will work either. (Timothy C. Hain, 2019)

Medications for nausea and vomiting:

Treatment of motion sickness differs from treatment of nausea and vomiting. A discussion of the treatment of vomiting can be found in this article. (Hain, 2020)

TIPS FROM CHAPTER 8

- Don't take any medication or pharmaceuticals for seasickness without first consenting your doctor!
- Scopolamine patches work for some people, but not for all. They require a prescription and can be expensive. For me, they caused severe headaches that were worse than the seasickness.
- Be sure the cure is not worse than the sickness
- Some antihistamines can help with seasickness and motion sickness, but you should consult a doctor before taking them.
- Some serotonin-based anti-nausea drugs have been known to help sufferers of motion sickness and seasickness, but definitely consult a doctor before using them.
- Migraine medications have been known to help with motion sickness, but please be sure to consult a doctor before using them.
- Some seizure medications may help with motion sickness, but you should consult a doctor before using them.
- The treatment for nausea and vomiting is different that the treatment for seasickness. Consult a doctor and research extensively before using any medications.

- Calcium channel blockers may be helpful in preventing seasickness, but consult a doctor before using them.

CHAPTER 9

Battling Seasickness the Natural Way

I am much more comfortable recommending natural methods that may help you battle seasickness. Pharmaceutical remedies simply do not work for me, but they may work for you. It's important to only try them with the recommendation of your doctor.

In this chapter, I want to address motion sickness in addition to the more specific seasickness as many of these behavioral methods and tips may help you.

- If you are riding in a car, sit in the front seat or drive.
- If you are on a ship, try to remain toward the middle of the boat and look at the horizon. Try to avoid tight spaces where you can't see the horizon.
- If you tend to get motion sickness on an airplane, ask for a window seat toward the front of the plane. Others recommend getting a middle seat.
- Face leeward. This way, if you vomit, it gets blown away from the ship rather than into it.
- Eat bland foods (crackers, bread, bananas, rice, applesauce, toast, etc.)
- Try to anticipate the motion. Drivers of cars and helmsmen of ships suffer less from motion

sickness or seasickness because they have a sense of balance and control.

- Anything with ginger can be very helpful for sufferers of seasickness and motion sickness. Try ginger tea, powdered ginger capsules, ginger candy, ginger snaps, ginger ale, even raw ginger between the teeth has a very soothing effect.
- Try peppermint to prevent seasickness. While sailing, I often would simply dab a little toothpaste on my tongue and found it very helpful in quelling the nausea.
- Many professional mariners suggest putting an earpiece or earplug in your non-dominant ear to provide balance. (If you are left-handed, place the earpiece in your right ear.)
- One sailor friend suggested drinking chocolate- or vanilla-flavored Ensure before setting sail to provide additional vitamins in case you get queasy and can't eat anything during a long passage.
- Place ginger tea, water, bananas, crackers, and other seasickness supplies in the cockpit for easy access while sailing. If you have to go down into the cabin to retrieve supplies, it could be uncomfortable, or the loss of fresh air could be detrimental. Easy access is important.
- Try devices like wrist bands or sea bands.

- Wear loose, comfortable, weather-appropriate clothing. Avoid tight clothing.
- Don't try to cook in rough conditions. Instead, prepare in advance some snacks and cold meals and have them available to grab and eat quickly in the cockpit.
- When you begin to feel uneasy, try to distract your brain with something that requires concentration (recite the Greek Alphabet, count to 100 in German, sing or recite the lyrics of your favorite songs, recite the dialogue from your favorite movie). Distractions help!
- One of my sailor friends recommends eating a large meal before departure, then quickly drink a can of Coca-cola in one gulp. Then burp. Different things work for different people, so perhaps the tip here is to find what works for you and do that!
- Fool yourself into believing you won't get sick. Say "I do not get seasick!" ten times before departure. Remember that seasickness is partly psychological so trick yourself into believing it won't happen to you. Mind over matter can be very powerful.
- Avoid strong smells like perfume, some food, sweaty crew members, diesel tanks, etc.
- Some people believe that chewing gum or sucking on hard candy can be effective against seasickness.

- Avoid dairy, alcohol, and anything that may make you feel bad on land. If it upsets your tummy on land, it will most definitely upset it at sea.
- Carrot juice, apricot juice, parsley, sage, rosemary and many other herbs and plants have been known to help with seasickness.
- Aromatherapy has been known to help people avoid seasickness. Use a fine mist sprayer with distilled water, lemon oil, cedar wood oil, dill oil, lavender oil, and a few drops of spearmint. Spray it lightly on your face.
- Adjust the sails and/or change the course. Sometimes a ship will get into a harmonic rhythm that can cause queasiness.
- Avoid books and computer screens.
- Lie in a hammock. This can greatly quell the motion.
- I know one sailor who swears that immersing your feet in ice water will stop the seasickness.
- Clean your ears with Q-Tips. Wax buildup can throw your system off balance.

CHAPTER 10

Do Animals Get Seasick?

Yes. After 12 full months of sailing in heavy offshore conditions with two beagles, Cap'n Jack and Scout, I can confirm that dogs do experience some level of seasickness, but perhaps not in the same way that humans experience it. I have definitely noticed that the dogs have been uncomfortable at times.

There was only one time that Cap'n Jack actually vomited, and it was a brief episode. On one passage, I noticed Scout struggling to get comfortable and actually threw up several times. Dogs have a very low center of gravity and fantastic balance. This helps them when conditions get rocky.

From my experience, and from talking to other sailors who sail with dogs, dogs seem to innately adapt to the conditions. For example, when Scout was battling seasickness, she stayed in the cool air and refused to eat anything. When we reached our destination and conditions became more calm, we noticed that she snapped out of the uneasiness quickly, just as humans usually do.

I found this information at **HOW CAN WE HELP OUR SEASICK DOG?** (Becker, 2012):

"Dogs get motion sickness when the inner ear gets jangled, causing nausea and dizziness. Motion sickness is more common in puppies, and many dogs outgrow it in part because they enjoy being out in the car—or boat, in your case—so much.

But the feeling of being sick may worsen over time into fear with similar symptoms, as the animal learns to associate being on the boat (or in a car) with discomfort. If you are boating on a lake or river and your dog is hanging his head over the rail in rough weather only, the occasional solution may be one of the motion-sickness medications people take. Just discuss it with your veterinarian first, because not all over-the-counter medications are safe for pets (some, in fact, are lethal), and you need to know if the drug is right for your dog and what the proper dosage will be.

For more severe or frequent cases, your veterinarian can provide a prescription medication that will help your dog. The same is true when anxiety is in the mix.

Because your dog only sometimes gets motion sick, however, I would want to know if you are boating on a saltwater body. Thirsty dogs will drink salt water (or take it in while swimming), setting up a cycle where they get thirstier (because of the salt) and drink more and more. If you're not paying attention, the first time you notice there's a problem may be when your dog throws up.

If the problem might be salt water, the solution is to make sure your dog is offered plenty of cool fresh water while you're out on the boat so that he's never tempted to drink the salty stuff."

DOGS AND MOTION SICKNESS (Flowers, 2018) is another helpful article. According to this article, dogs don't turn the unflattering shade of green that people do when they're experiencing motion sickness, but there are some signs of dog travel sickness you can learn to identify. These include:

- Inactivity, listlessness, uneasiness
- Yawning
- Whining
- Excessive drooling
- Vomiting
- Smacking or licking lips

The best way to prevent dog travel sickness, according to the article, is to make the atmosphere as comfortable as possible for your dog, keep him in the fresh air, give him plenty of water, and limit his food intake.

For further research, read this fascinating article: **DO ANIMALS GET SEASICK?** (Eveleth, 2012).

100 TIPS FOR BATTLING SEASICKNESS

Here is a recap of my 100 Tips for Battling Seasickness that will help you Get Your Sea Legs! If you found this book and these tips helpful, please consider leaving a review on Amazon or Goodreads.

1. Strap yourself securely in the cockpit to prevent yourself from falling out of the boat. (Or to prevent throwing yourself overboard, which may be what you feel like doing.)
2. Stay away from areas with strong smells, like the locker containing the diesel tanks. Avoid other strong smells like perfume, sweaty crew members, pungent food, etc.
3. Try to eat something, even if you throw it back up. Try to digest some calories.
4. Remember that the effects of seasickness most likely will not stop until the motion stops, so accept this and try not to panic.
5. Don't watch the clock. Try to focus on something else, if at all possible, so you don't focus on how much time is still left to go on the passage.
6. If possible, lie flat on your back in the cabin and try to sleep (sometimes this is not possible if you are sailing with a small crew).
7. After a bout with seasickness, get back out there as soon as possible so you don't lose your nerve later. You don't want this to be your last-ever memory of sailing.

8. Understand the history of seasickness and know that it happens to the best of us. At least you can know that you are in good company. Some of the world's greatest sailors and seamen have experienced seasickness.
9. If you have recently had changes in your eyesight (new glasses, lasik surgery, new contact prescription, etc), you may be more susceptible to seasickness.
10. If you are a migraine sufferer, you may be prone to seasickness and might wish to avoid any situation in which extreme motion occurs.
11. If you are a woman, take precautions as research shows you may be more susceptible to seasickness and motion sickness than men, especially during your menstral cycle.
12. Do not go below deck for extended time periods, unless it is to sleep.
13. Do not look through binoculars for long periods of time.
14. Do not stare at objects your brain will interpret as stable. Anything that involves staring at one point such as reading a book, staring at a computer screen, doing detailed needlework, or even staring at a compass might bring on a bout of seasickness.
15. Try to relax and not focus on your fears. The anxiety of fear can greatly contribute to seasickness.
16. Keep something on your belly and consider the reverse tastes of food (for example, an apple or

banana tastes a lot better coming back up that tuna or yogurt).

17. Try to keep a stable temperature and dress appropriately for the weather. Extreme cold and extreme heat can contribute to seasickness.
18. Stay hydrated! Hydrate well the day before and the morning of departure. This means avoiding alcohol and also taking at least a few sips of water, even during heavy bouts of vomiting. Hydration will also help to prevent muscle cramps.
19. Try to stay on deck in the fresh air and focus on anything other than the moving ship.
20. Take deep breaths and control your breathing rhythm.
21. When on deck, facing forward (rather than to the side) seems to help most people.
22. Remember that you need to let your brain adjust to this new unstable environment by allowing the horizon to act as the true point of reference.
23. Try to eat, but avoid spicy, acidic, or fatty food. Eat bland foods (crackers, bread, bananas, rice, applesauce, toast, etc.). Avoid dairy, alcohol, and anything that may make you feel bad on land. If it upsets your tummy on land, it will most definitely upset it at sea.
24. If possible, cruise in relatively calm waters.
25. Nerves, excitement, and fear can contribute to seasickness. Try to stay calm the day of departure.
26. Try to get a good night's sleep the night before departure.

27. Take a good shower before departure so you feel refreshed.
28. Eat well the night before departure.
29. Avoid alcohol the night before departure and during the passage.
30. If you choose to take seasickness medicine, it's best to take it about two hours before departure. Once the seasickness sets in, it's too late.
31. Try to avoid medicine that will make you drowsy if you know you have a shift at the helm within 6 hours.
32. When you begin to feel queasy, stay busy. Grab the wheel, to feel a sense of control, or focus on a small task.
33. When conditions get rough, reef the main sail and adjust the sails in a way that cushions the motion.
34. Stay in the fresh air, if possible.
35. Try not to focus on the queasiness. Find anything else to focus on!
36. Lie flat in the center part of the ship with your eyes closed. Try to sleep, if possible.
37. Rest when you can, even if you don't feel tired.
38. Either stand up or lie flat on your back when you feel the seasickness set in. Don't sit.
39. Hold a potato in your left hand. Sometimes mind over matter works if you truly believe it.
40. Try not to let fear paralyze you.
41. Don't feel bad about succumbing to the seasickness and trust the rest of the crew will help

you with the sailing responsibilities. This kind of anxiety can make the seasickness worse.

42. Trust your captain to alleviate the fear that you may be in danger.
43. Trust your ship to get you to your destination safely.
44. Trust yourself and try to reassure yourself that everything will be Ok.
45. Remember: "The brave one is not the one who has no fear. The brave one is the one who has fear… but does it anyway."
46. Embrace the things you love about being on the water and try to focus on the good things rather than the queasiness or the fear.
47. Arm yourself with information but try to avoid doing too much research about bodies of water or conditions that scare you.
48. Try to enjoy the journey by focusing on the good parts and think about the excitement of the destination rather than the difficulty of the passage.
49. Mentally prepare for challenging passages so you can be prepared and quell the fear.
50. Don't take any unnecessary chances with the weather or conditions. Wait patiently for the perfect weather window before departing.
51. When you see huge waves headed your way, try to brace yourself before contact to prevent excessive movement.

52. When captain and crew are seasick, shorten the shifts (for example, from four hours to two hours).
53. Find a comfortable place in the cabin to sleep—one in which you won't be tossed around too much (for example, on the floor between the bunks).
54. Don't try to cook in rough conditions. Instead, prepare in advance some snacks and cold meals and have them available to grab and eat quickly in the cockpit.
55. Prepare a thermos of ginger tea before departing and keep it handy in the cockpit in case the queasiness sets in.
56. When you feel the uneasiness set in, try to distract yourself with something that requires concentration (for example, recite the Greek Alphabet, count to 100 in German, sing or recite all the lyrics of a song, recite dialogue from your favorite movie). Listen to an audible book or music. In other words, distract your brain.
57. Challenge yourself. (For example, I made it a goal to never miss a shift, no matter how bad I felt). This will give you something to strive for and a happy feeling of accomplishment.
58. Find something to hold on to for balance (for example, a winch drum).
59. Stress can be a psychological trigger for motion sickness. When in a provocative motion situation, try to relax and not think about stressors like your job.

60. Try not to think about past bouts with seasickness when you are on a boat or in a situation that causes extreme motion.
61. Try to fight the feeling rather than surrendering to it so quickly.
62. Some studies show that visuospatial training can help quell the effects of motion sickness.
63. Don't take any medication or pharmaceuticals for seasickness without first consulting your doctor!
64. Scopolamine patches work for some people, but not for all. They require a prescription and can be expensive. For me, they caused severe headaches that were worse than the seasickness.
65. Be sure the cure is not worse than the sickness
66. Some antihistamines can help with seasickness and motion sickness, but you should consult a doctor before taking them.
67. Some serotonin-based anti-nausea drugs have been known to help sufferers of motion sickness and seasickness, but definitely consult a doctor before using them.
68. Migraine medications have been known to help with motion sickness, but please be sure to consult a doctor before using them.
69. Some seizure medications may help with motion sickness, but you should consult a doctor before using them.
70. The treatment for nausea and vomiting is different that the treatment for seasickness. Consult a

doctor and research extensively before using any medications.

71. Calcium channel blockers may be helpful in preventing seasickness, but please consult a doctor before using them.

72. Spread your legs shoulder-width apart, bend your knees, and perform a slow-motion, hula-hoop action with the lower part of your body to cushion and balance the movement.

73. Carefully plan your passage. Try to determine just the right time for departure to best take advantage of the weather, wind, currents, and conditions. Then determine the best route, remembering that the conditions could change at any time at sea.

74. Remember that it's the hard parts of sailing that make it special. If it were easy, anyone could do it.

75. Delay the departure if you are feeling rushed, or stressed, or if you have other injuries that are bothering you.

76. Sometimes mind over matter is the best cure. Try not to think about the queasiness, if possible. Try to focus on the beauty surrounding you—the sunset, the colors, the scenery, etc. This will help to take your mind off of the uneasiness.

77. Remember that seasickness is not your fault. Don't get mad at yourself or frustrated when it sets in. Instead, focus on ways to quell the effects. Frustration will only make it worse.

78. Try to keep your sense of humor and find ways to relax and laugh with other crew members.

79. At times when you are feeling ok, try to cook something to have a warm, substantial meal in your belly, if at all possible.
80. Try not to squint at the sun. This could cause a headache, which could lead to seasickness.
81. Sometimes taking an antihistamine will help to clear the sinuses and help you to avoid seasickness.
82. Try to avoid having a pity party and focusing on all the ways you feel bad. Try to find something positive to think about. Physical discomfort can creep into your psyche and make you convince yourself you feel worse.
83. Face leeward. This way, if you vomit, it gets blown away from the ship rather than into it.
84. Try to anticipate the motion. Drivers of cars and helmsmen of ships suffer less from motion sickness or seasickness because they have a sense of balance and control.
85. Anything with ginger can be very helpful for sufferers of seasickness and motion sickness. Try ginger tea, powdered ginger capsules, ginger candy, ginger snaps, ginger ale, even raw ginger between the teeth has a very soothing effect.
86. Try peppermint to prevent seasickness. While sailing, I often would simply dab a little toothpaste on my tongue and found it very helpful.
87. Many professional mariners suggest putting an earpiece or earplug in your non-dominant ear to provide balance. (If you are left-handed, place the earpiece in your right ear.)

88. One sailor friend suggested drinking chocolate- or vanilla-flavored Ensure before setting sail to provide additional vitamins in case you get queasy and can't eat anything during a long passage.
89. Place ginger tea, water, bananas, crackers, and other seasickness supplies, snacks, and drinks in the cockpit for easy access while sailing. If you have to go down into the cabin to retrieve supplies, it could be uncomfortable, or the loss of fresh air could be detrimental. Easy access is important.
90. Try devices like wrist bands or sea bands.
91. Wear loose, comfortable, weather-appropriate clothing. Avoid tight clothing.
92. One of my sailor friends recommends eating a large meal before departure, then down a Coca-Cola in one gulp. Then burp. Different things work for different people, so perhaps the tip here is to find what works for you and do that!
93. Fool yourself into believing you won't get sick. Say "I do not get seasick!" ten times before departure. Remember that seasickness is psychological so trick yourself into believing it won't happen to you. Mind over matter can be very powerful.
94. Some people believe that chewing gum or sucking on hard candy can be effective against seasickness.
95. Carrot juice, apricot juice, parsley, sage, rosemary and many other herbs and plants have been known to help with seasickness. This book includes 101 plants that may help you.

96. Aromatherapy has been known to help people avoid seasickness. Use a fine mist sprayer with distilled water, lemon oil, cedar wood oil, dill oil, lavender oil and a few drops of spearmint. Spray it lightly on your face.
97. If possible, lie in a hammock. This can greatly quell the motion.
98. I know one sailor who swears that immersing your feet in ice water will stop the seasickness.
99. Clean your ears with Q-Tips. Wax buildup can throw your system off balance.
100. Whether it's the challenge or the joy of sailing, the scenery or the wildlife, remember why you do this so you will know that the bouts with seasickness are worth it!

Works Cited

A. Lawther, M. G. (1988). *Motion Sickness and Motion Characteristics of Vessels at Sea*. Retrieved from Pub Med: https://pubmed.ncbi.nlm.nih.gov/3208731/

al, G. e. (1996). The Vestibulo-Ocular Reflex and Seasickness Susceptibility. *Journal of Vestibular Research*.

Beck, J. (2015). The Mysterious Science of Motion Sickness. *The Atlantic*.

Becker, M. (2012, May 18). *How Can We Help our Seasick Dog?* Retrieved from Vet Street: http://www.vetstreet.com/dr-marty-becker/how-can-we-help-our-seasick-dog

Benson, A. (1999). *Aviation Medicine*. Oxford, UK: Butterworth-Heinemann.

Boater, D. (2018). *4 Common Travel Disorders and How to Manage Them*. Retrieved from Dan Boater: https://danboater.org/travel-health-and-safety/4-common-travel-disorders-and-how-to-manage-them.html#motionsickness

Bob Cheung, K. H. (2001). *Lack of Gener Difference in Motion Sickness Induced by Vestibular Coriolis Cross-Coupling*. Retrieved from Pub Med: https://pubmed.ncbi.nlm.nih.gov/12897401/

Bunting, E. (2016). *What are the best remedies for Seasickness?* Retrieved from Yachting World: https://www.yachtingworld.com/features/feeling-rough-take-edge-off-seasickness-survey-76032#HKhv8msohOPGZwJt.99

Crislip, K. (2019). *Motion Sickness Prevention and Cure Tips*. Retrieved from Trip Savvy: https://www.tripsavvy.com/motion-sickness-prevention-and-cure-tips-3149753

Dobie, T. G. (2019). *Psychological Mechanisms That Exacerbate Motion Sickness*. Cham Springer.

Dornhoffer, J. (2004). Stimulation of the Semicircular Canals Via the Rotary Chair as a Means to Test Pharmacologic Countermeasures for Space Motion Sickness. *Otology & Neurotology.*

Erskine, S. K. (2019). Motion Sickness CDC Guidelines - Travel By Air, Land & Sea. *Traveler's Health,* Chapter 8.

Eveleth, R. (2012, May 14). *Do Animals Get Seasick.* Retrieved from Life Science: https://www.livescience.com/33771-animals-seasick.html

Flowers, A. (2018, May 15). *Dogs and Motion Sickness.* Retrieved from Pets WebMD: https://pets.webmd.com/dogs/dogs-and-motion-sickness#1

Furman, J. D. (2011). Rizatriptan Reduces Vestibular-Induced motion sickness in migraineurs. *The Journal of Headache and Pain.*

Garrison, L. (2019, July 16). *How to Avoid an Treat Seasickness.* Retrieved from TripSavvy: https://www.tripsavvy.com/how-to-avoid-and-treat-seasickness-992029

Grunfeld, G. (1999). Relationship Between Motion Sickness, Migraine, and Menstruation in Crew Members Around the World Yacht Race.

Guru, M. S. (2021). *A Brief History of Motion Sickness.* Retrieved from Motion Sickness Guru: https://www.motion-sickness-guru.com/a-brief-history-of-motion-sickness.html

Hain, C. (2020). *Dizziness and Balance.* Retrieved from Dizziness and Balance: https://dizziness-and-balance.com/index.html

Huzar, T. (2020). Can we ease motion sickness through mental training? *Medical News Today.*

Jeffrey Wisch, M. (2021). *Safety and Seamanship.* Retrieved from SAS Cruising Club: https://sas.cruisingclub.org/node/257

Knox GW, W. D. (1994). Phenytoin for Motion Sickness: Clinical Evaluation. *Laryngoscope 104.*

Konrad, J. (2016, June 1). *What is Seasickness? And 50 Ways Professional Mariners Tackle It!* Retrieved from GCaptain: https://gcaptain.com/seasickness-ways-tackle/

Lee JA, W. L. (1986). Calcium antagonists in the prevention of Motion Sickness. *Aviat Space Environ Med.*

Russell, J. (2017). *The Atlantic Crossing Guide, 7th Edition.* New York: Bloomsbury Publishing Plc.

Schmal. (2013). Neuronal Mechanisms and the Treatment of Motion Sickness. *Karger.*

Segrest, M. (2018, 2019, 2020, 2021). *How to Get Your Sea Legs.* Retrieved from Navigate Content, Inc.: www.navigatecontent.com/sailing-adventure-blog

Shupak, D. e. (1994). Cinnarizine in the Prophylaxis of Seasickness. *Clin Pharmol Ther.*

Timothy C. Hain, M. (2019, June 7). *Motion Sickness.* Retrieved from Dizziness-and-Balance: http://www.dizziness-and-balance.com/disorders/central/motion.htm

About the Author – MICHELLE SEGREST

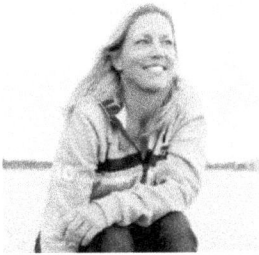

Michelle Segrest has been a professional journalist for more than 30 years. She is the president of Navigate Content, Inc., a full-service content creation firm, and works hard for her clients even while sailing the world.

Michelle is a proud Southern girl from Sweet Home Alabama. She sailed for the first time with a longtime friend in Hamburg, Germany in 2013 and was immediately hooked. Sailing became a part of her soul as this journalist found a passion that would burn deeply within her forever. She still delights in researching and learning the finer details of sailing.

In 2018, she embarked on a year-long sailing adventure that included an Atlantic Crossing with passages across the Baltic Sea, the North Sea, the English Channel, the Bay of Biscay, around the Atlantic coast of Spain and Portugal, around the western coast of Africa and across the Atlantic to Brazil and then up the South American coast.

She chronicles her adventures in her award-winning blog, "How to Get Your Sea Legs." Be sure to read her sailing memoir, **"Living Life Sideways."**

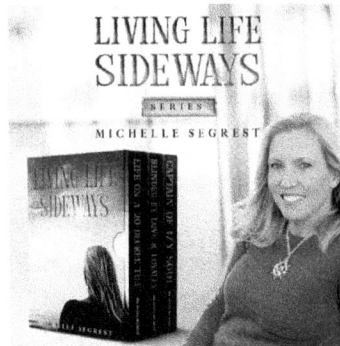

Books by Michelle Segrest

LIVING LIFE SIDEWAYS
True Story of Heart-Pounding Adventure & Heart-Wrenching Survival

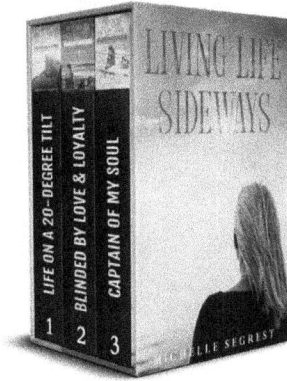

"A very impressive testimony of grit, determination, and a journey toward self-valuation."

If you thought sailing the world is an endless holiday of bikinis and martinis, get ready for a bucket-list adventure of a lifetime!

These gripping true stories open a window into the liveaboard lifestyle and complex challenges of blue water sailing—where simple decisions have real-life consequences and where the most provocative obstacles live inside a sailor's soul.

If you are intrigued by an escape from the ordinary, come aboard as a sailor and two seadogs discover exactly what it's like to live life sideways.

CAPTAIN'S LOGBOOK & JOURNAL FOR SAILORS

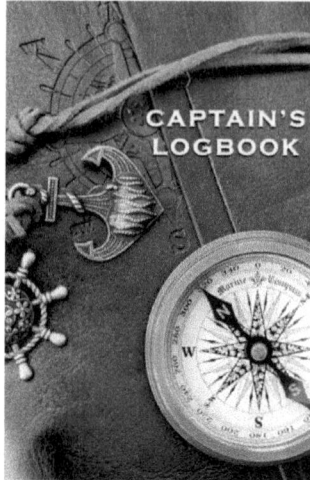

HOW TO SAIL WITH DOGS
100 Tips to Help You Get Your Sea Legs

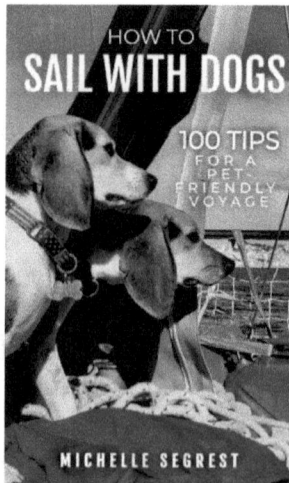

CAP'N JACK & SCOUT'S
TRAVEL ADVENTURES
Childrens Book Series

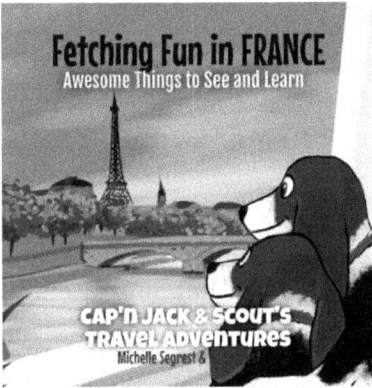

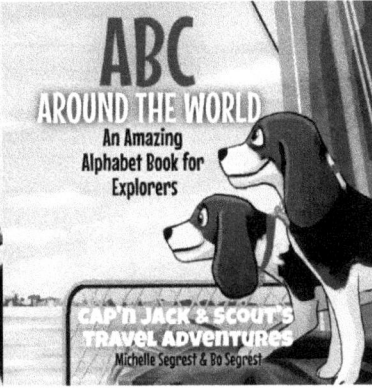

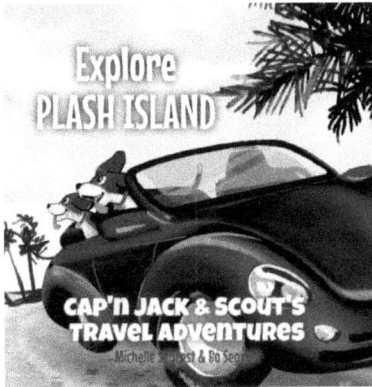

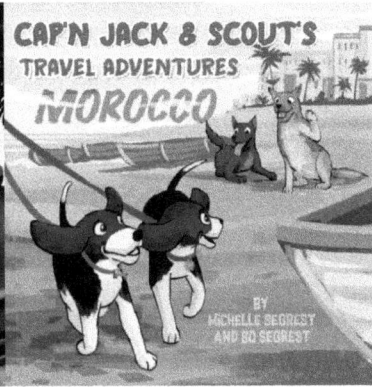

www.ingramcontent.com/pod-product-compliance
Lightning Source LLC
Chambersburg PA
CBHW071232020426
42333CB00015B/1441